A HAPPY HEALTHY YOU

A WOMAN'S GUIDE TO HAPPINESS, HEALTH & HARMONY

Mary Johanna McCurley, J.D. | Jyotsna Sahni, M.D.
Jan DeLipsey, Ph.D. | Lu Jurcova Phillips, M.S. | Kristi McIntyre, M.D.

Copyright © 2010 Mary Johanna McCurley, J.D.
All rights reserved.

ISBN: 143926449X
ISBN-13:9781439264492
Library of Congress Control Number: 2009911648

A HAPPY HEALTHY YOU:

A WOMAN'S GUIDE TO HAPPINESS, HEALTH AND HARMONY

TABLE OF CONTENTS

Preface .... **vii**

Part One: The Second Half of Your Life Can Be Better Than the First Half 1

    Chapter 1: Successful Aging: A New Model for Growing Older 3

    Chapter 2: Change Your Life: Choose Joy 11

    Chapter 3: Optimism's Main Ingredient: Reclaiming Hope 27

Part Two: A Moving Experience 47

    Chapter 4: With the Wind in Your Hair: What Aerobics Is All About 49

    Chapter 5: Curling Iron: Strength Training 65

    Chapter 6: These Heels and Hills Are Killing Me: What Women Do That Makes Their Bodies Hurt 93

Part Three: Food for Thought: Nutrition **113**

    Chapter 7: Your Mother Was Right After All: Food for Life – Mindful Eating 115

    Chapter 8: Chocolate Is a Major Food Group, Isn't It? Healthy Weight Strategies 131

Part Four: **What You Don't Know May Kill You** **153**

    Chapter 9: The Good, the Bad, and the Ugly:
                Menopause – The Heat Goes On 155

    Chapter 10: Bust Your Butt, Not Your Hip:
                 Bone Up on Osteoporosis 185

    Chapter 11: How to Stay Young at Heart:
                 Women and Heart Disease 201

    Chapter 12: Every Woman's Worst Fear: The Ticking
                 Time Bomb – Breast Cancer 215

    Chapter 13: What's Sleep Got to Do with It? 229

Part Five: **You Are What You Think:**
                The Mind-Body Connection **253**

    Chapter 14: The Heart and Soul of Any Woman:
                 Relationships 255

    Chapter 15: Your Personal Pathway to Peace and
                 Tranquility 265

    Chapter 16: Take the Words "I Can't" Out of Your
                 Vocabulary: The Road to Change 271

Acknowledgments **277**

PREFACE

by

Mary Johanna McCurley, J.D.

When I first considered writing this book, the title was to be Fat, Dumb, and Not So Happy, until we realized that it was a bit of a downer and might not exactly fly off the shelves. And ultimately, it wasn't the life-affirming message we wanted our book to convey. This book is about how you—yes, you—can live a happy, healthy, and harmonious life, regardless of where you are now or what's happened before.

Whether you're well into menopause or still in college, if you're a woman, this book is for you. Women have made unbelievable strides in recent years. And although that progress was hard-won and we don't know many women who want to go backward, we still find ourselves asking, "Is that all there is?" I believe that our Creator wants us to be happy, joyous, and free, but the rest of the world, sometimes including me, often seems dead set against it. This book is intended to be a guidepost to improving the quality of our lives.

Part of the problem is physical. Obesity is an epidemic in America, and the diseases that accompany it are crippling us and our health-care system.

But our problems aren't entirely physical. We have unrealistic expectations of what our lives should be, what we should look like, and how our homes should look. We fail to appreciate the extraordinary beauty that surrounds us, or celebrate the daily miracle of life.

That's where Fat, Dumb, and Not So Happy came from. Many women—more of us than we care to admit—are living in an unhealthy and unhappy state, and most are at a loss regarding how to get off that treadmill.

Let's look at fat. Sixty-two percent of all women in the United States between the ages of twenty and seventy-four are overweight, and about one-half of that population are actually obese. A direct correlation exists between body weight and deaths from all causes in women. Additionally, women who are obese appear to be subject to more prejudice and discrimination than their male counterparts. Research shows that obesity affects every aspect of a woman's life—from financial support, to college attendance, to job opportunities, to social relationships.

Next, there's dumb, because women haven't taken control of their lives. We blame our weight, health, and moods on others: our parents, our jobs, our children, and our spouses. We're "dumb" because we've let society convince us that being in charge of our own lives is impossible.

And generally, we're not so happy because throughout history women have tended to be unhappy about a lack of choices in their lives. In the twenty-first century, however, we have so many choices that we're overwhelmed. We're depressed, we're anxious, and we feel "less than"—less than our expectation of ourselves, or less than the expectations others may have of us (real or imagined).

We have seen the enemy and she is us. The good news? We all have the opportunity and means to create positive changes in our lives. That's the purpose of this book.

This book is by five women, all with different backgrounds and areas of expertise. And it's about our individual journeys to find balance and happiness in our lives. We want to share our experience, education, and hope with you, and we hope you will share it with the women in your lives.

Let's meet each of the women contributing to the book.

Preface

KRISTI MCINTYRE, M.D.

Dr. Kristi McIntyre is an attractive forty-something physician who specializes in oncology and, even more particularly, breast cancer. I met Kristi at a neighborhood restaurant my husband and I fondly call "the fish place." The fish place is much like the bar in *Cheers*, where everybody knows your name. Many of us eat there several times a week. I don't know if that means we have no imagination, or if we all come to get a healthy meal, or if the food takes a backseat to the sense of community we feel there. I will say this: it's always nice to meet my neighbors and be able to talk to them, not hampered by the labels and confines of our respective careers.

To see Kristi with her beautiful, energetic four-year-old daughter and prince of a husband, no one would guess that she is a busy doctor who deals with the pain that breast cancer brings to so many women. Kristi is a bit shy, but she is a whiz of a doctor who is consistently named one of Dallas's best. You too will think she is the best when you see how her analytical mind works. You will be equally impressed by all the heart that's behind it.

JYOTSNA SAHNI, M.D.

I met Dr. Sahni during my annual visit to Canyon Ranch in Tucson, Arizona. I had seen another female doctor there for several years and was irritated that my usual doctor wasn't going to be there during one of my visits. I don't know if Dr. Sahni could sense that I was less than pleased, but if so, she didn't let on. She is a beautiful woman with an East Indian background. She has more education than seems possible for such a young woman. She is Board-Certified in Clinical Nutrition, Geriatric Medicine, Holistic Medicine, Internal Medicine and Sleep Medicine. Had I known all of her qualifications at the time of our first encounter, I admit I would have been a bit intimidated.

What caught my attention was her comment that she'd always thought it would be so cool if they made broccoli in a pill. (I agreed, because while I like broccoli fine and wouldn't mind benefiting from it, I wouldn't want to eat it every day.) She went on to explain that, lo and behold, such a pill actually does exist now, and she thought that with my mother's history of colon cancer, I should consider taking it. WOW! A classically trained medical doctor pushing health food supplements for preventive medicine. How refreshing! I've been sold on her ever since, and in the chapters ahead I believe you will be too.

LU JURCOVA PHILLIPS, M.S.

Lu's real name is Lucie, but because Americans pronounce it like Lucy of *I Love Lucy* rather than the beautiful pronunciation of her native language, she shortened it to Lu. She is anything but short. Lu came to this country from the Czech Republic to attend undergraduate school on a volleyball scholarship. She got her master's degree in exercise physiology and has been in the United States ever since.

Lu was recommended to me as a strength trainer, and we hit it off immediately. She is young, pretty, and very smart. She actually makes working out fun, and in her beautiful Czechoslovakian accent she explains what she's asking you to do and the reason for doing it. Working out with Lu is never a task; it's something to look forward to. She understands that strength training does not come naturally to most people, so she has made it something joyful and playful. I know that in the chapters ahead you will be motivated by her jubilant, caring spirit.

JAN DELIPSEY, Ph.D.

Of our group of five, I have known Dr. Jan DeLipsey the longest. She and I are, in many ways, very much alike, and in many

Preface

ways we are quite different. Jan is a petite and attractive forensic psychologist who spends most of each day trying to help people understand other people's motivations, as well as their own. No, she doesn't have a crystal ball, although I know that some days she wishes she did. What Jan has is a gift for understanding human nature and a desire to help individuals draw the best out of themselves to reach their potential.

I had known Jan for many years when we found ourselves working on a case together in Phoenix, Arizona, on September 11, 2001. For those of us over fifty (which Jan and I are), there are certain days and events in the history of our nation that are burned into our brains: where you were when John F. Kennedy was shot; where you were when the Beatles were on Ed Sullivan; where you were when the first man landed on the moon; and, of course, where you were on September 11, 2001. We were trapped in Phoenix, could not fly home, and all cars had been rented. Our generous client loaned us her car, and a group of us started the long drive back to Dallas. We talked for hours over that two-day period in the car (as everyone in our country did) about what the attacks meant for our nation and how they would change our lives forever. What was different for us was that we were together in the back of a car for many hours over the course of two days.

What I learned about Jan in those hours I will carry in my heart for the rest of my life. I got a glimpse of her great inner strength, her deep sense of caring, and her ability to pass on her uplifting spirit to others. I know that Jan will help you on your journey as she and all the authors of this book have done for me.

MARY JOHANNA MCCURLEY, J.D.

I am a family law attorney as well as a personal and executive coach. As you may have guessed, the coaching grew out of my work as a divorce lawyer. Seeing so many clients in emotional pain, wondering what went wrong with their lives and their marriage, inspired me to look for ways to help them do more than just end their marriages.

Over the years, I have come to know my co-authors, both personally and professionally, and they have helped me find health, happiness, and harmony in my own life. I know they will do the same for you.

This book is about more than possibilities. It is about making life choices that make us younger than our years and help us, with each new day, to look forward to what life has to offer.

It's time to celebrate the fact that we're in charge of our own lives. It is within our control to be happier, healthier, and more in harmony with our world—more this year than last, and next year even more than this year. So let's get started.

Preface

A NOTE FROM PSYCHOLOGIST JAN DELIPSEY:

Millions of women in the forty-years-plus phase of life are afflicted by unhappiness and an array of health problems. Life doesn't have to be this way. Health, longevity, and happiness can be had by most of us. What's the secret?

This question is the real reason we, the women who wrote this book, gathered together. We decided we were not going to stand by and watch the women we love, women who are in a position to have terrific lives, just flat miss the boat. Enough. We decided to stand shoulder to shoulder and offer women something better. That is how this book, which is for women by women, came about.

As you read these pages, it won't take long to realize that this is not your run-of-the-mill "get fit" kind of book. It's a guide to a better and healthier life and it's from the heart. We have had a world of life experience, literally: medicine, psychology, law, finance, nutrition, exercise physiology, horse training, art, music, teaching, lecturing, nurturing, researching, and mothering. I could add partners, lovers, and friends, but you get the picture. We bring more than two centuries of combined life experiences, failures, and successes to the table. Our shared core value is that we care what happens to the women in our families, the women who are our friends, and the women we serve in our professions. We juggled careers, families, and responsibilities to lock arms and write this book—not such an easy task when you are living life to the fullest already! So, as you read this compilation of knowledge, research, and thought, remember that it is sincerely from the hearts of women who have made this journey with success. We are a group of gloriously happy and healthy women, and we have included in this book the personal stories of many, many gloriously happy and healthy women. We invite you to join us. Use this book as a guide to a better life. We did it for you.

Disclaimer

The workouts and exercises presented in this book are merely suggestions and do not represent the full range of exercises available to work individual body parts. If you have any injuries or conditions that prevent you from doing any of these exercises safely or comfortably, *please do not perform them.*

If you would like to develop a weight-training regimen, we highly recommend that you consult with a personal trainer. Even if you can't see the trainer on a regular basis, one or two sessions will allow you to get started on a workout that you can periodically update with your trainer (every six to eight weeks).

The best workout is the one tailored to your body and its needs. Nevertheless, the sample workout in this book provides a good overview of the body parts that should be worked on a regular basis.

PART ONE

THE SECOND HALF OF YOUR LIFE
CAN BE BETTER THAN THE FIRST HALF

CHAPTER 1

SUCCESSFUL AGING: A New Model for Growing Older

Thoughts from Mary Jo:

It's been said that you know you're getting old when you do more things for the last time and fewer things for the first time. Have you thought any new thoughts lately? Dreamed any new dreams? Set any new goals? Taken any new action?

If you pay attention, there are women all around us who inspire us and are seemingly forever young. Is it just better genes? Of course, good genes help, but if you examine these women's lives more closely you will see that it is far more than just good genes.

While running in a race a couple of years ago, I noticed a woman who was more than a decade older than I. Some of us were running a 5K, some a half marathon, and others an entire marathon. You could tell how far someone was running by the color of the number displayed on her shirt. Martha, the older woman, was running a marathon. As if that were not remarkable enough, I noticed that she had a joyous look on her face. (I was having trouble just breathing.) Martha intrigued me so much that I sought her out after the race and asked if she would mind telling me how old she was. She proudly told me it was her seventieth birthday *that day*. I asked her how many marathons she had run; she said it was her first.

I asked with amazement, "Why did you decide to run a marathon at the age of seventy?" She responded, "Why not!"

Why not, indeed? It is in this spirit that we say to you, "Why not?" Why not feel younger, act younger, and in many cases look younger? It is yours for the taking.

We're not telling you to run a marathon (unless that's what you want to do). But we are saying, why not start taking a yoga class, or start a walking club with some friends, or plant that garden you've always wanted?

The purpose of this book is to get the word out that, as women, we do not have to accept a negative, limiting model for aging. Yes, our hair may gray (that's easily taken care of) and our skin may wrinkle, but we don't have to accept the maladies that our mothers accepted.

We all have mothers or someone we love who, just as their children were all grown and they could finally take some time for themselves, were suddenly faced with failing health. Whether it was heart disease, stroke, breast cancer, osteoporosis, crippling arthritis, or the inability to get around like they used to, they found themselves sentenced to watching daytime TV in an easy chair.

A large percentage (if not half) of all illnesses and injuries that occur after forty can be prevented. Half! The great thing is that whether you fall prey to these illnesses or injuries is within your control. In large part, YOU decide if life after forty is to be better than the first forty years—or worse. Hear me again: it can be much, much better or it can be much, much worse.

Experts on aging say that as many as 70 percent of early deaths can be avoided. If death is too hard for you to relate to, then let's talk about quality of life. Do you want to need assistance getting out of your chair and walking—or do you prefer doing it under your own steam?

I'll take a story from my own life. My grandmother fell and broke her hip at the age of seventy-three. For all practical purposes, she didn't get out of the house again until thirteen years later, when she died, mainly because she was tired of living a life in which she was totally dependent on others.

But as sad as my grandmother's story is, it's not what made me decide to write a book about health issues for women. It hit me like a bolt of lightning one day when I was listening to a lecture on aging. The speaker made the remarkable statement that those of us in the room who make it to age sixty have a better-than-even chance to make it to a hundred. Wow! Am I—are any of us—prepared to live that long? I don't want to be my grandmother, trapped within four walls and alive but not really living. Do you? I suspect not, or you would not be reading this book.

I decided right then and there that the message had to get out to women that we can lead happy, healthy, and harmonious lives well into our eighties and possibly our nineties, if only we make the right choices.

I am saddened when I see fellow co-workers and friends making choices that will harm their chances of a healthy life. Frankly, death is not the scary part—it's the total dependence on others (whether it be doctors, loved ones, or hired assistants) that scares the living daylights out of me. It's the constant pain of joints and muscles, or the inability to walk, or being unable to play with my god-children that I don't wish to face.

About the same time I decided such a book needed to be written, I was having chronic neck pain, so I went to my chiropractor. I asked her, "Why is my neck doing this?" She said, "I hate to tell you this, but you're just getting old."

I WON'T ACCEPT THAT, AND NEITHER SHOULD YOU!

So you may ask, "What does a lawyer have to offer about living a healthy and happy life?" What I have is my own experience of aging and how I have dealt with it, as well as twenty-nine years of coaching women. More importantly, I am blessed to have access to some of the finest experts to help us successfully navigate this path we are going down. It didn't make sense to keep their knowledge under a bushel, so I brought them together to share their wisdom with you and me.

The truth is that we have become a society that accepts heart attacks, cancers, strokes, and broken bones as a normal part of aging. Our Western culture has decided if a pill or surgery doesn't fix it, you have to accept it as a part of life. Having been to such places as India, China, and Japan, where many of the people DON'T accept such cultural norms, I have to wonder why Americans are willing to settle for less than the best.

When I see what life can be, I get mad. Mad because our society treats disease *after* you are sick, instead of teaching us how to prevent broken bones, heart disease, or things as small as aches and pains. The world around us says, "It's simply a part of growing old." Well, ladies, WE ARE BEING LIED TO.

In my career as a lawyer I have felt passionate about issues such as the rights of children, protecting an abused spouse, or helping my profession deliver ethical, quality service to the public. All of those issues I felt were within my power to change, so I took leadership positions in my field to work on them.

But how could I effect change in the lives of women about their health? How could I let my sister, my female friends, my female clients know about this LIE, this MYTH, this CON, that we must accept that the last third of our lives must be filled with pain, misery, and unhappiness?

It was clear at this moment in the lecture that I had to bring together some of the best women's health issue experts to help tell the truth to women.

So Where Do We Start?

Our bodies were designed to catch that saber-toothed tiger and eat it—or maybe to run from it or be eaten ourselves. Our predecessors would store up fat because they didn't know when their next meal might be coming. Our bodies have not adjusted to eating constantly, much less a steady diet of McDonald's and Taco Bell, lounging in an easy chair, and driving everywhere. There is a big difference between real aging (which is natural, and otherwise called "primary aging") and the unnatural process of the body breaking down (called "secondary aging").

The broken bones, sore joints, and lack of balance are not symptoms of natural aging—things atrophy from lack of use. I still remember the day I looked in the mirror and saw wrinkles. I had looked younger than my age my whole life, and it seemed like overnight I had grown old. However, while I am not happy about the wrinkles, the occasional gray hair that sticks out in a funny way, or the way gravity has affected certain parts of my body—those things are all a natural part of aging. BUT, while you may look your age, you don't have to accept negatives or limitations as a natural part of aging.

The most important anti-atrophy thing you can do for yourself is movement. (We are going to talk a lot more about movement in part 3.) I'm not saying you have to be chased by a saber-toothed tiger, but you might want to pretend to be.

If you get nothing else from this book, let it be that you MUST get off the couch and move. If you don't, it won't matter what you eat, what self-help book you read, or what pill you take, because you are going to experience negative, not positive, aging.

Take heart, though, because even minor changes can make a difference, according to many studies. For example, an overweight smoker who cuts back on snacking and loses a small amount of weight can significantly reduce the risk of cardiovascular disease.

I'm not going to pretend that I understand everything I've studied about this topic, or everything my fellow authors have told me, but it boils down to this: our bodies are hardwired through millennia of evolution to walk miles to find food. And when we found food, it was usually fruits and nuts. Now we simply walk to the refrigerator and find a bounty of high-calorie meats, cheeses, sweets, and processed foods.

This lack of activity tells your body that there is no food to hunt, and therefore it begins to store fat in order to survive. Early man had no reason to be sedentary, unless there was no food and he or she had to save energy. Our bodies respond to this threat by grabbing on to every calorie.

Other factors are, of course, important, such as what you put in your mouth. Is it a Big Mac, a cigarette, and a Coke? Or is it salmon, nuts, and water?

Equally important is staying engaged in your community and living a balanced life. A study by Rotten and Stephenson (2000) indicates that stress can accelerate the aging process and that healthy long-term relationships can slow it. Your body thinks that if there is no movement and no interaction with the world, you are settling down to die. This is not "primary aging" but "secondary aging." It's not caused by your genes or unavoidable changes, but by YOU. Everything you put in your mouth; every movement (or lack thereof) in a day; and whether your outlook is positive or negative—all affect whether your body, mind, and spirit stay young. With proper nutrition, movement, and engagement in life, every woman can embrace a new model for aging that is dramatically different from the one our grandmothers followed. In the next few chapters we will explore "staying young forever" and what that really means.

I recently had the good fortune to meet Florence Rink, who is ninety-four years young. I had the opportunity to observe her and her habits for a week. I also had the privilege of interviewing Florence.

My observations were that she would walk all over the several-hundred-acre campus we were on and that she always had a smile on her face.

Florence was born in 1914, and as soon as she could, she took up ballroom dancing. She danced the tango and the twist and everything in between. Before Florence married, she went to work for Sears and became the first woman credit manager the company ever had. When she married, she had to keep it a secret because women who were married were not allowed to work. Those were tough times, but she didn't let it get her down. Florence and her husband had a daughter, and the family often traveled. She has been on more than fifty cruises, and she plays bridge, gardens, and goes to the theater. In other words, she stays engaged.

Regarding her diet, Florence follows some simple rules: she avoids sugar, white flour, and processed foods, and eats almonds every day.

When asked her secret to staying young, she said, "Keep moving, eat properly, have a positive attitude, and live every moment." Her parting words to me were, "Tell those young women to keep dancing."

CHAPTER 2

CHANGE YOUR LIFE: Choose Joy

A merry heart doeth good like a medicine.
—*Proverbs 17:22*

Thoughts from Mary Jo:

Abraham Lincoln once said: "Most of us are as happy as we decide to be." Nike has another way of saying it: "Just do it!" In Alcoholics Anonymous, they say: "Fake it until you make it." Before you dismiss these sayings as trite, let's analyze them.

We can't make the mistake of letting our life circumstances dictate whether or not we are happy. Life is always going to be full of challenges, and if we wait until everything is perfect at home or at work or with our health, happiness will never come. Instead, we can choose to be happy in all circumstances. Happiness truly comes from within, not from external forces.

Happiness is more than a feeling; it's a way in which you see yourself. It's a state of mind. According to Dr. Dan Baker, a clinical psychologist and author of several books regarding happiness, research shows that "happier people are more hard-working, more socially engaged, and healthier than those who are less happy."

If we are constantly asking, "Why can't I be taller, smarter, thinner?", or "Why can't I have a better job, better house, better spouse?" we will never be happy.

Remember Kermit, the little green frog on *Sesame Street*? He sings the following song: "It's not easy being green, having to spend each day the color of grass when I think it would be nicer to be red or yellow or gold or something much more colorful even than that. It's not easy being green, you seem to blend in with so many ordinary things and people tend to pass you over because you're not standing out like flashing sparkles in the water or stars in the sky."

Then he changes his tune *after making a decision to be happy* and sings "but green, after all, is the color of spring and green can be cool and friendly or big like an ocean or important like a mountain or tall like a tree. When green is all there is to be, it could make you wonder why, but why wonder? I'll do fine. Green is beautiful and that's what I think I want to be."

What is it you think you want to be? Is it something near to what you really are? Because if you listen, you can hear the little green frog's song in the bank, in the post office, in the hair salon, in the school. "It's not easy being me."

While in China doing some research for this book, I met an eighty-five-year-old woman who, even though she lived in a very humble home with few conveniences, seemed to be quite happy. She shared her secret to happiness:

1. Be grateful for what you have

2. Never compare yourself to others

3. Stay active and engaged in life

When I am grateful for the many blessings I have, when I quit trying to be like someone else, and when I stay engaged in life, the tune in me (like that of the little green frog) begins to change.

Look at your "green"—all the experiences you've had, all the sunrises you've seen, all the friends you've made, all the people you've loved—and you'll see a balanced new view of yourself. Then you can say, "Yes, I am green and I like it fine; it's what I'd like to be."

Ralph Waldo Emerson understood this when he said: "What lies behind us and what lies before us are tiny matters compared to what lies within us." So, what can you do to find joy?

1. Make sure you find joy in your movement. Learn to play again. Remember when you were a kid walking down the street? One block you might skip, the next play hopscotch, and the next run full-out. You weren't exercising—you were having fun and enjoying life. I try to duplicate that playfulness in my aerobic work. If I'm inside, I walk for a few minutes and then lift weights for two, then run for five minutes, then do another set of weights for two. If I'm outside, I run as hard as I can to a certain landmark, then I walk or skip to another, and so on. Try to remember where you found joy as a kid in movement and duplicate it.

2. Find ways to laugh a lot. After a stressful week at work, I like to go to a movie—preferably a comedy, even if it's a silly one. Laughter is good for your immune system. It produces endorphins (natural painkillers) and decreases levels of stress hormones. Martin Luther instinctively knew that when he said: "If you're not allowed to laugh in heaven, I don't want to go there."

3. Lastly, spend time with friends who have a positive outlook on life. All of us have friends who are always complaining or have something wrong in their lives. I'm not saying that you should no longer spend time with those friends, but limit how much time you do spend with them.

I still remember the slumber parties I went to as a kid. Everyone would laugh and tell stories until all hours of the night. Pick a day each week or month to get together with your girlfriends, and have lunch or dinner or go to a movie together.

Above all, be mindful of all that is around you and look for the joy in everything you do, whether it be cooking, working, or playing with your grandchildren.

CHANGE YOUR LIFE: Choose Joy

What the Psychologist Has to Say: Jan DeLipsey, Ph.D.

The Big Three: Beliefs, Language, and Choices

Are you satisfied with your life? Let's start by taking a little inventory. Read the five statements below and score each one using a scale from 1 (strongly disagree) to 7 (strongly agree).

1 – Strongly disagree; 2 – Disagree; 3 – Slightly disagree; 4 – Neither agree nor disagree; 5 – Slightly agree; 6 – Agree; 7 – Strongly agree

____ **In most ways my life is close to my ideal.**

____ **The conditions of my life are excellent.**

____ **I am satisfied with my life.**

____ **So far I have gotten the important things I want in life.**

____ **If I could live my life over, I would change almost nothing.**

____ **Total**

Now, take your total score and compare it to the categories below.

35 – 31	Extremely satisfied
26 – 30	Satisfied
21 – 25	Slightly satisfied
20	Neutral
15 – 19	Slightly dissatisfied
10 – 14	Dissatisfied
5 – 9	Extremely dissatisfied

Did your score fall where you thought it would? Let me help you put your score into perspective. The average score for the middle-aged to older American women is about a 26 (two points below that for men.) In other words, most American women are on the lower end of "satisfied" with their lives. That's not what I would call particularly impressive, given the state of world affairs and the war-ravaged places where we could be, but are not, living. College students, prison inmates, hospital patients, abused women, and other groups score even lower.

Your score on this Life Satisfaction Scale probably is a good reflection of your level of optimism in life. If your score falls into the "Slightly Satisfied" category or lower, you have some room to grow. If your score falls into one of the higher categories, then let's see what you can do to accentuate the positive. Let's see what we can do to change our lives and find a higher level of satisfaction.

Beliefs, language, and choices are the fundamental keys to a better life. Once you get these keys in place you can unlock your personal obstacles to exercise, nutrition, stretching, being involved in the world in a meaningful way, happiness, and all the rest of the "goodies" you want in your life. I'll come back to these fundamental keys later in the chapter. For now, just know that the goodies come naturally when you have the keys in place.

I can already hear differing versions of "Yeah, but…" creeping into your mind right now. You are rationalizing and thinking that I don't understand where you are in your life. Maybe you're living with and taking care of an elderly parent, unexpectedly raising your grandchildren, have had to go back to work because your retirement plans fell flat, or are having serious health problems. No doubt, this stage of life brings challenges—hard challenges. As my eighty-six-year-old mother (who shares a home with me) is fond of saying, "Getting old isn't for sissies." But quite frankly, what is the alternative? Give up? Continue living a life fraught with depression and illness? Walk around with a resentment chip on your shoulder? Be a pain in the behind to people who love you? Die early? Die poorly? I don't want this for my life, and I know you don't either.

The good news is that once you get the hang of managing your beliefs, language, and choices (the fundamental keys), the rest comes naturally. I didn't invent these concepts, although I did come up with my own personal version of how to understand and incorporate them. These conceptual principles of living come from a solid and lengthy history of social science research in what is popularly known as "positive psychology." You are probably familiar with psychological research as it relates to problems such as depression, anxiety, or trauma. How could you not be, with antidepressant ads on television every hour on the hour?

With antidepressant medication being the most widely prescribed drug in America, it looks like we are all pretty good at being depressed. What the women in our country really need is more education in learning how not to be depressed. But I'll wager you aren't so familiar with research in the positive psychology movement because it just hasn't received the popular attention that it should. This is a shame, because it's this positive stuff that really makes life more doable and enjoyable. Positive psychology researches and promotes positive events and experiences, such as understanding and teaching "success," "optimism," and "life satisfaction."

The Good News

Because you are still reading and have made it this far into the chapter, I suspect you have that one thing no one can give you—the desire, the hope to improve your life. Even if your hope is small and wavering, the fact that it is there is enough. This small flicker is all you need to turn your life around.

As I was finishing this chapter I had the good fortune to spend time with Dr. Robert Maurer, the author of *The Kaizen Way – One Small Step Can Change Your Life*. After talking with him and reading his work, I returned to this chapter because I just hadn't given enough consideration to how frightening or overwhelming change can be for many people. For a lot of women change invites fear—even if it is a change that obviously will be for the better. It can be fear of the unknown, fear of failure, and, sadly, even fear of success.

Fear is definitely public enemy number one when it comes to change. Fear, as you probably well know, is a powerful and debilitating emotion. If, like me, you have had a history of failed diets, relapses to fast-food chains, workout routines that went bust, and periods of despair when you just gave up and didn't care anymore, this different approach to change will intrigue you. It works.

When I am afraid, I can feel it physically, in my gut. Sometimes this visceral reaction is so strong I can't even think clearly. Dr. Maurer makes a profoundly persuasive argument that fear has deep physiological roots that inhibit change. When I first heard this slant on fear, it made a lot of sense to me. When my gut would seize up with fear, there was no doubt that it felt like a deep physiological root taking hold.

Let's look at the mechanics of fear. When a woman makes a change or faces a change that causes her fear factor to kick in, her abilities to reason and to think logically and creatively go by the wayside. What a bummer. Just when you need to be clear-minded and on your toes, your survival mode takes over and starts interfering with rational thinking and creative problem solving. Ever mentally freeze up in a crisis or before taking a test? You're not alone. It's human nature to freeze in a crisis. All your energy and resources are focused on surviving the perceived threat. This is a normal human response; emergency workers have to undergo special training to switch into active rather than reactive mode in a crisis.

If you are in a fear or crisis mode, the important "big three"—beliefs, language, and choices, which are all higher-order cognitive activities—have a tendency to shut down. This is terrific if a huge lion is chasing you across the African plains and your brain says, "Feet, don't fail me now." You have to get out of there and run for your life. It's not so terrific if your fear is keeping you from positive change, such as exercising more or improving your diet.

Looking back at the times when I wanted to change something in my life and "failed" (what I now affectionately refer to as "learning opportunities"), I now realize there was a common thread: I took on too much, too fast, with little or no confidence. Significantly, I failed to shift my beliefs, language, and choices. Conversely, when I did dive headfirst into deep water and made a huge and lasting change with success, I had no fear and no doubts about what I had to do or my ability to do it. My big three—beliefs, language, and choices—were aligned with my positive intentions.

Comparing my successes in change versus my "learning opportunities," the differences come down to my own confidence. Or, as Dr. Maurer might put it, whether or not the fear factor had taken over. I have been more successful in making lasting changes in exercise, practicing good nutrition, or taking a risk in a relationship when I didn't feel overwhelmed. When I have been able to keep my language, beliefs, and choices in operational mode, I have done well and been highly successful in achieving the changes I wanted.

Keeping the Fear Factor under Control

How do you keep your fear factor under control when you are ready to make a change? Simple: take a small step instead of a giant leap. When the fear factor is roused, the best way to combat it is to take "baby steps." Find a step to change that is so small that the fear factor does not kick in. Let me tell you how I reached this conclusion.

How do you make a first step? Decide. Just decide. Decide to have a better life. Visualize it. That's enough for the first step. If you need time to contemplate and talk to others about this decision, take it. Take an hour, take a day, take a week, take a nap, take a trip. Take what you need in order to know that you can be unshakable and unfaltering in your decision. It might take days for some or only five minutes for others. Don't worry about the second step at the beginning. One step at a time is enough.

I finally learned to battle fear successfully by taking a "one day at a time" approach. In the past, when some of my warp-speed lifestyle changes failed, I usually drew back to a kinder, gentler, more realistic path that set me up for success (i.e., small steps). I just stumbled on this "chunk it down" recipe for change, and it worked. There's a second piece to this. For the first couple of decades of my career, I was a part of the recovery journey of thousands of women and girls who overcame devastating, traumatic events—kidnapping, rape, and other violent abuses. I have personally witnessed these survivors meeting their fears head-on in small doses, bit by bit, and returning to normal, if not better, lives. Let me introduce you to a few of them.

Kim: Home Alone

Years ago, I counseled a woman who had been abducted by a stranger and held hostage for more than fifteen days. For all intents and purposes, the odds that she would survive this ordeal had been extremely low. However, she was smart, a fighter, and very lucky.

When I met Kim, she had yet to be alone and was living with her sister. Though it had been only about six months since the ordeal, she wanted a therapist to help her take her life back. She wanted her independence back (I told you she was a fighter). We set her first goal: to come straight home after work and spend thirty minutes alone before her sister got home. On her first attempt, she completely lost it after a few minutes and had to call for help. She was a basket case. I convinced her that this was merely a learning opportunity (rather than a mistake), and we went back to the drawing board.

During this time I had been studying therapy through allegory, so our next try at being alone centered around a metaphor of physical rather than emotional healing. We imagined we were a team helping a woman learn to walk again after having survived a near-fatal car accident. Working from this perspective, we reasoned that we would want our imaginary patient to just stand first and get her balance, then take a step or two, not run around the block. Kim and I then set her next goal, visualizing being alone for only five minutes for several days, and then actually trying it. It worked! Bit by bit she increased her time alone. I saw her only a few more times after that because she was well on the road to recovery. She got her life back—five minutes at a time.

In those early years of my clinical work, I learned from the successes of my clients, like Kim, what worked and what didn't. Then I used this experience, along with the excellent professional training I received at a women's university in Texas, to guide other women to better, more satisfying lives. I learned firsthand that one step at a time, even a very small one, was a surefire way to overcome whatever life throws at you.

Imagine how excited I was this past year to find Dr. Maurer and his work about using small steps to neutralize the brain's fear response. He studied, explained, and actually published a book about the physical and psychological mechanisms underlying successful change. I learned through him that there really is social science research to back this up. But when I stop to think about it, don't these ideas about change fall into the common sense category too? The mantra of Alcoholics Anonymous, "One Day at a Time," has guided millions of people to overcoming alcohol and drug addiction through a step program. Small steps have proven to be the way to walk down a path of change.

Willa: "It's Never Too Late"

I first noticed Willa because every time I was on the track at my health club, she was already there, slowly but very surely making her way around the loop. Unconventional in her choice of workout clothing (preferring jeans and a long-sleeved T-shirt to the traditional gym attire), she caught my eye the first day I was there. Willa was as thin as a rail and a bit humped over, but she moved around that track at the speed of light. My interviews with Willa, except for the one when I insisted on sitting down to review my notes with her, were all on the track while we were walking. She wouldn't slow down, not even for me.

At seventy-one, Willa had been a smoker and had advanced osteoporosis and vascular problems in her legs. Her physician told her to get her affairs in order. She did, but not in the way he meant. Willa had that flicker of hope, a desire for a healthier and longer life. So when she heard this pseudo-death sentence from her doctor, she started walking. Step by step, she walked away from death's door. She is still walking today, at age eighty-two.

During one of our discussions, Willa shared a heartbreaking story about her dear friend who had bad knees and was overweight. Willa told me that her friend thought she was too old to change her life, too old to work out. Increased pain from increased weight and increased weight from lack of activity eventually left her friend a lonely and depressed invalid. I commented that her friend sounded like she didn't try to save herself as Willa had. Still walking, Willa looked me straight in the eye and pronounced with unrestrained authority, "It's never too late; it's just never too late."

"Yes, I believe you" was my verbal response, but my mental note to myself was "wondrous things happen when you decide to take that first step."

How was it that Willa had a flicker of hope, which her friend did not? How was it that Willa was able to get her feet moving, when her friend could not? Willa simply decided. She decided that it was not yet time to die. She had a will to change her life. She took a step, then another one, and then another one. And quite frankly, the steps got easier and easier with time. She is still going strong.

Elizabeth, the Reformed Pessimist

Elizabeth was divorced. Her husband had run off with a younger woman, her one adult child lived overseas, and Elizabeth was bitter, very bitter. She habitually described her life as "awful." She was obsessed with complaining about her thirty-plus-year marriage ending in disaster, and could (and often did) recall slights and bad behavior by her husband from the day they first met. If nothing else, Elizabeth's ability to recall and cite this lengthy and detailed list of wrongdoings was an impressive exhibition of memory. Elizabeth rarely had anything positive to say about anyone. She was predictable in her amazing ability to put a negative interpretation on just about any event. Her favorite words were "worst," "awful," and "terrible." People avoided her. Elizabeth felt bad. She struggled with depression and could not understand why she was so miserable.

Elizabeth and I took a short therapeutic journey together. After we had a few sessions, I congratulated her for being the most professional pessimist I had yet to encounter as a psychologist. I told her that happiness was beyond her reach and that she shouldn't waste any more money on therapy. Rather, she should just accept the natural consequences of her self-imposed world of negative thought and language and remain miserable. Over the next two hours, Elizabeth tried to convince me that she really could and did want to change her life. Somehow, during her soliloquy about change, she had a moment of clarity that changed her life forever. She accepted responsibility for her own happiness and well-being. She decided—she just decided—to be different. Elizabeth had that spark that I talked about earlier: the desire to have a different life. She went on to pursue a new life and her own dreams. She learned to look forward with hope rather than back with resentment. She became a completely different person—a happier and more satisfied person—and it started with a conscious decision. She just decided.

What really happened to Elizabeth? She picked up the mantle of personal responsibility. She made the decision to have a different life. From there, I helped her learn how to live optimistically by changing her language and her view of the world. Then, as if by pure magic, people were drawn to her and her life was full.

What We See and What We Say: Language and Beliefs

Let's look a little closer at this change in Elizabeth. What we see informs what we say and what we say informs what we see. I'm talking about language—what we say, and beliefs—what we see. Remember when I told you I would return to the fundamental keys in more detail? Well, here we are.

When I first met Elizabeth, she used fatalistic language. She complained about everything, even me, the shrink who was trying to help her. Her spoken language was highly negative and pessimistic. In like manner, Elizabeth rarely missed an opportunity to interpret an event in the most negative light possible and to expect the worst. Her outlook was extremely gloomy. She was stuck in what I call a "negative feedback loop," with her world view and her language feeding off each other in a highly efficient negative way. Gloom and doom spawned more gloom and doom, and so forth. This intensely negative approach to living limited the opportunities (choices) available to Elizabeth.

Elizabeth's experience of life was a very lonely one. Her reality testing was right on: no one wanted to be around her. When I first met her, Elizabeth was not consciously aware of how her negative approach to living was impacting her life. To me, how she got to where she was really didn't matter so much. Maybe her ex-husband was really a stinker; maybe he was overwhelmed by Elizabeth's negativity; maybe her father was abusive. There comes a point, though, when it truly doesn't matter. What was important when I met Elizabeth was helping her get on and stay on a different road of life, a positive and fruitful one. I showed her the way, but she took the steps.

World view and language are interdependent, and they exist in a fluid state. There is a lot of psychology research to back me up here. Said another way, language continuously reflects and shapes what you believe (your world view), and what you believe continuously reflects and shapes your language.

For example, if a committed pessimist loses her job, she will say things like, "This is the worst possible thing that could happen. This is the worst day of my life. I'll never get over this, and I will end up on the street with nothing. I am an idiot. Why couldn't I just hold on to my job like everyone else?" Obviously her language about the job loss is extreme, and has taken a form of monumental pessimism. This language feeds a world view that she is a failure. She sounds like the queen of hopelessness: it totally colors her world view. She will soon slip into depression (who in her right mind would not, with this world view?) and will continue in a downward spiral. Eventually our unemployed pessimist will become so overwhelmed that she won't even be able to look for a new job. She'll be so depressed and desperate no one will want to hire her or, for that matter, even be around her. Her fears, fueled by her language, will eventually become her reality. She suffers—not so much from losing her job, but from her *world view and language* about losing her job. Because of this negative lifestyle, the doors and opportunities available to our unfortunate pessimist are probably going to slam shut—over and over again.

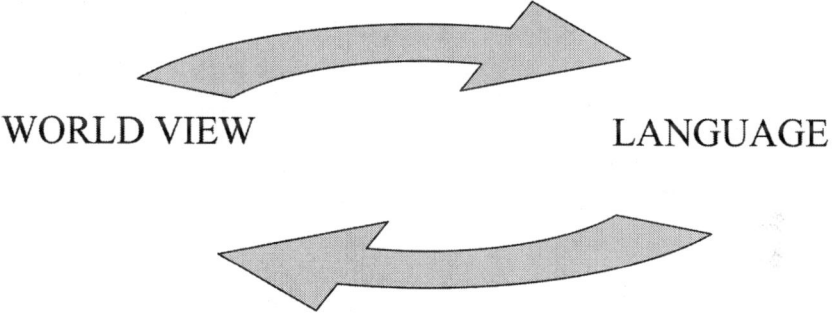

WORLD VIEW   LANGUAGE

Now let's look at how a committed optimist might view losing her job. "This is a challenging day but I will get through it. It's probably not the best day of my life, but it certainly isn't the worst. I need to get creative and start looking for another door to open. Who knows—maybe this is a blessing in disguise! The more doors I knock on, the greater the chances that I can land another job. Rejection just means that I haven't knocked on enough doors." This language reflects a world view that is both optimistic and more balanced. Our optimist acknowledges that being unemployed is plenty stressful, but appropriately places this unwanted event in a context of hope and change, not catastrophe and disaster. This woman will spiral upward toward the stars! Staying in an upbeat emotional mode supported by positive language will inspire her to actually find a new job and, in the process, make her more attractive to potential employers. Furthermore, she doesn't even have to really believe it in the beginning. Doing the "fake it till you make it" thing really works. If you say it enough and don't let yourself wallow in negative emotions, pretty soon your world view will get on board with your optimistic language. It's a win-win.

This language/world view discussion is not a new one. It has been the subject of centuries of philosophical debates. But the aspect we are interested in here is a bit more practical. Language and world view are directly tied to whether a person approaches life from an optimistic or a pessimistic perspective. And this, my friends, is what it's really all about. The optimistic woman finds life better, more meaningful, happier, satisfying, *and* she enjoys the benefits of being healthy and living longer. Not a bad deal if you can get it. And by the way, you *can* get it.

CHAPTER 3

OPTIMISM'S MAIN INGREDIENT: Reclaiming Hope

But a broken spirit drieth the bones.
—*Proverbs 17:22*

Thoughts from Mary Jo:

Lucille Ball once said: "One of the things I learned the hard way was it doesn't pay to get discouraged. Keeping busy and making optimism a way of life can restore your faith in yourself."

I know it is easier said than done. We have to cultivate optimism. Why do it? It is very simple: optimistic people live longer. You need to do it for you!

I do a simple exercise at the beginning of each day. It takes only five minutes. Write down what you are grateful for that day and an amazing thing will happen: it changes your entire day and your attitude toward it.

I know some days you don't feel grateful about anything. On those days, your list might look like this:

1. I am grateful that I can walk.
2. I am grateful that I can talk.

An example, from a recent newspaper column:

Dear Abby:

Happiness is knowing your parents won't almost kill you if you come home a little late on Saturday night. Happiness is having your own bedroom. Happiness is having parents who trust you.

Happiness is getting the telephone call you've been praying for all day. Happiness is getting good grades and making your parents proud of you. Happiness is being a member of a popular crowd. Happiness is having parents who don't fight. Happiness is knowing you're as well-dressed as anybody. Happiness is something I don't have. Fifteen-year-old Unhappy Girl.

Next to it was printed:

Dear Abby:

Happiness is being able to walk, to talk, to see, to hear. Unhappiness is reading a letter from a Fifteen-year-old Unhappy Girl who can do all of these things, and still isn't happy. But I can talk, I can see, I can hear. I just can't walk. Fifteen-year-old Happy Girl.

The simple, meaningful, valuable things had become real to her.

Helen Keller, the first deaf/blind person to earn a Bachelor of Arts degree, said it so well when she said: "Optimism is the faith that leads to achievement. Nothing can be done without hope and confidence."

As I said earlier, we have to cultivate optimism. At the age of ninety, Regina Brett wrote the following "45 Lessons to Live By," published in *The Plain Dealer* (Cleveland, Ohio). Put them by your bed or on your desk and read them every day.

1. Life isn't fair, but it's still good.
2. When in doubt, just take the next small step.
3. Life is too short to waste time hating anyone.
4. Your job won't take care of you when you are sick. Your friends and parents will. Stay in touch.
5. Pay off your credit cards every month.
6. You don't have to win every argument. Agree to disagree.
7. Cry with someone. It's more healing than crying alone.

OPTIMISM'S MAIN INGREDIENT: Reclaiming Hope

8. It's OK to get angry with God. He can take it.
9. Save for retirement starting with your first paycheck.
10. When it comes to chocolate, resistance is futile.
11. Make peace with your past so it won't screw up the present.
12. It's OK to let your children see you cry.
13. Don't compare your life to others. You have no idea what their journey is all about.
14. If a relationship has to be a secret, you shouldn't be in it.
15. Everything can change in the blink of an eye. But don't worry; God never blinks.
16. Take a deep breath. It calms the mind.
17. Get rid of anything that isn't useful, beautiful, or joyful.
18. Whatever doesn't kill you really does make you stronger.
19. It's never too late to have a happy childhood. But the second one is up to you and no one else.
20. When it comes to going after what you love in life, don't take no for an answer.
21. Burn the candles, use the nice sheets, wear the fancy lingerie. Don't save it for a special occasion. Today is special.
22. Over prepare, then go with the flow.
23. Be eccentric now. Don't wait for old age to wear purple.
24. The most important sex organ is the brain.
25. No one is in charge of your happiness but you.
26. Frame every so-called disaster with these words, "In five years, will this matter?"
27. Always choose life.
28. Forgive everyone everything.
29. What other people think of you is none of your business.
30. Time heals almost everything. Give time.
31. However good or bad a situation is, it will change.
32. Don't take yourself so seriously. No one else does.
33. Believe in miracles.
34. God loves you because of who God is, not because of anything you did or didn't do.

35. Don't audit life. Show up and make the most of it now.
36. Growing old beats the alternative—dying young.
37. Your children get only one childhood.
38. All that truly matters in the end is that you loved.
39. Get outside every day. Miracles are waiting everywhere.
40. If we all threw our problems in a pile and saw everyone else's, we'd grab ours back.
41. Envy is a waste of time. You already have all you need.
42. The best is yet to come.
43. No matter how you feel, get up, dress up, and show up.
44. Yield.
45. Life isn't tied with a bow, but it's still a gift.

OPTIMISM'S MAIN INGREDIENT: Reclaiming Hope

What the Psychologist Has to Say: Jan DeLipsey, Ph.D.

By the time you're forty, you know with certainty that no one escapes hard times. Bad and tragic events do not discriminate. They happen to everyone, and to some more than others. There are some problems you cannot do much about. Nevertheless, if you cannot change the problem, then you can change the way you look at it and its impact on your life. I am not discounting the harsh realities of poverty, illness, or other serious tragedies of life. But if you give in when you encounter these kinds of adversities, you give up any hope of overcoming them.

We walk for cancer survivors; we fight for them and treat cancer even though there is no cure. Many women (the optimists and the survivors) find ways to live well in spite of having faced a cancer diagnosis. These women have hope. Without hope, problems are insurmountable. We have to find a way to sustain hope, be optimistic, and approach life positively, regardless of the nature of the problems we face. Being optimistic doesn't mean being naive or blessedly oblivious to the pain and suffering that life will bring. Rather, optimism meets life's curve balls head-on, with hope and with purpose. As Grandma Moses said, "Life is what we make it, always has been, always will be." So, make it as good a life as you can.

More about Optimism and Pessimism

Returning to the example of the woman who lost her job, the pessimistic woman jumps to the worst possible scenario. In other words, she lets her mind go to all kinds of possible bad outcomes. She ruminates and worries about all the possible catastrophic outcomes of even neutral events. Her language reflects the depths of her pessimism, and she is prone to depression, unhappiness, and all the other accompanying health problems of living in a chronic state of stress. She sees the negative event with permanence and as being insurmountable. When this negative feedback loop starts spiraling downward, it spawns a whole new host of negative problems—overeating, lack of exercise, withdrawal from social situations, poor performance at work, and stress in relationships. Things just get worse and worse and worse, in all aspects of living. Then, if she is like most women in America, she will find herself taking pills for depression and anxiety, thus relying on a pharmaceutical company to solve her problems rather than her own mind and heart.

Let's take a look at the factors underlying this pessimism: **fatalistic thinking** (worst-case scenario), **a sense of permanence** (it will never end), and **a feeling of no control** (insurmountable). Understanding these nasty little underlying factors will help you break the cycle of pessimism. Knowing these factors will make it easier for you to search and destroy harmful thinking and language habits.

Finally, on a more positive note, let's see what you can add to your quiver of life skills. The optimistic person jumps to the best possible scenarios **(hopeful thinking)** when faced with challenges. She sees a **bad event as temporary**, a normal part of life, but one that can be overcome **(controllable)**. She problem-solves; she doesn't fall into a rut of rumination. Her language is upbeat and solution-oriented. This helps her keep a positive world view. When her "positive feedback loop" finally begins spiraling upward, she inevitably comes out better rather than worse for having gone through the difficult experience. This is the person who rises above adversity and uses it to her advantage. She learns that she, not a publicly traded company, is in charge of her life.

Now look below; winning thinking patterns are on the right. The more you can live with the patterns on the right (the light side rather than the dark side of the force), the better off you'll be.

Fatalistic Thinking and Language	Hopeful Thinking and Language
Bad Event Is Permanent	Bad Event Is Temporary
Bad Event Is Uncontrollable	Bad Event Is Controllable

OPTIMISM'S MAIN INGREDIENT: Reclaiming Hope

What I am talking about here is very simple: you are in control of your thinking and language habits—what they are and how they are shaped. You can decide (like I have, and like the other women who wrote this book have) to be optimistic, happier, and healthier. Or you can decide to go down a darker road. To me, the choice seems like a no-brainer. But then again, I'm an optimist.

Echoes from Times Past

The language and world view that you live with, day in and day out, may be rooted in your distant past. Many times negative messages take hold in early childhood. Years and years of repetition ingrain them, and to some extent they are reinforced by life experience. Going back to my example in the previous chapter, Elizabeth was devastated that the people she loved avoided her. Her negative outlook on life was so alienating that it was true. From her brief reminiscences, though, I suspect her negativity was well in place by the time she married.

For Elizabeth, cynicism and pessimism were her way of coping with life—a mental defense that she believed shielded her from disappointment (she expected the worst from people and got it), but also trapped her in a rut of cynical rumination. In essence, by living in the dark side of the force (remember the habits on the left side of the thinking pattern diagram?) *she got what she gave*. Somewhere along the early road of life, Elizabeth learned to live and stay in the shadow lands and, through years of repetition, these patterns trapped her into decades of unhappiness.

Elizabeth changed her life without wading back through and re-defining painful experiences from her childhood. For Elizabeth, there may or may not have been clearly defined events that set her on a pessimist road. For many of us, though, there are very specific painful events or experiences that bleed into today's thoughts and language.

Of the thousands of girls I counseled who were violently abused by strangers or distant relatives, the ones for which I had the most concern had unstable families, fragile support systems. Rather than being strong and confident about their daughters' recovery, they were instead full of woe and gloom, often verbalizing that their daughters and families would never recover. Abuse that occurred within the family, of course, presented a rockier road to recovery. In the instances where family members stepped up as an advocate for recovery, the girls did pretty well. In these instances, it wasn't the nature and extent of the abuse that was most predictive of recovery. Rather, it was the meaning the family and others ascribed to the bad event. The child who recovered quickly was the child whose family blamed the true offender, supported her for reporting the abuse, and believed she would recover. The simple assignment of blame and shame was often the single most defining principle of which child remained a victim versus which child became a survivor.

Although these abuses are events we all agree are egregious, there are other, more subtly harmful experiences that can have equally devastating outcomes. What happens to the little girl who hears negative messages, day in and day out? "You always mess things up. You're weak. No way would I trust you with my car. You look like garbage; go wash off that makeup." Something as small as not being invited to the seventh-grade dance—for a child who has lived in this kind of a negative fog—can be absolutely demoralizing. Of course, it's not the lack of invitation; it's the meaning the girl (or sometimes others around her) ascribes to it. Not being asked to the dance is confirmation of all these negative messages. You can see where this is going: our histories as girls, for better or worse, echo into our present.

Why is it that one victim continues as a victim and the other becomes a survivor? Why is one person who grew up with negative messages able to re-program her beliefs and another is not? No one really knows. But what I can tell you is that people who recover from abuse and succeed are hopeful and optimistic. They

OPTIMISM'S MAIN INGREDIENT: Reclaiming Hope

choose to be survivors rather than continue to be victims. Their painful past inspires them, rather than defeats them. Although you cannot choose your childhood experience, and it is in the past anyway, you can choose how you look back on it now.

You can take past painful events and turn them around in such a way as to make your life better. This doesn't work in the abstract. You have to be purposeful and direct. Use the chart below and first write down the five most painful past events or messages from your childhood and your past inner dialogue about them. Actually write them down. Writing in and of itself is healing, plus it forces you to define exactly what happened and how you interpreted it. Now here's the hard part: go back and put the most optimistic spin on those events that you can.

Event or Message	My Past Language	My Current Language

These things are what they are, but even if they are long gone you might still be hearing their echo. Ruminating on the negative can trap you in the shadow lands. If you live there long enough, that's what you will become. Leave it!

If you could not reinterpret some of these bad events, then it's time for some serious soul-searching. Letting the past continue doing harm in your life today is a decision—a decision on your part that just continues the harm. Look in the mirror: the image you see today is your offender as well as your savior. Not exactly fair, but this view at least gives you a way to save yourself from the past cruel actions of others. It all starts with small steps.

Whatever you can do right now, right at this moment, take a positive step to start changing how you see and talk about these events. Put them in a different frame, even if it is a small one. You don't have to wait. You don't have to go through any rituals or years of therapy. You don't have to telephone or confront anyone about past transgressions or wrongs. If you want to, fine, but you don't have to. Take the harmful power of the past and reframe it (turn it) into something positive for yourself. You *can* change how your past negative experiences affect you today.

Make your mind, language, and beliefs focus on the things that will bring joy, peace, and a quiet sense of well-being to your life. Bad experiences don't have to be reinvented as happy occasions. Find a way to make them tolerable, though, and useful to you. Make the messages that were once rocks in your shoe, causing you to stumble, now cause you to jump higher.

I'm not saying that you can erase an abusive event. I am saying that you can find a way to stop it from ruining your life. Oprah Winfrey, one of my all-time favorite women, sometimes talks about the rape she suffered as a child. She has transformed a personal tragedy into a way to reach out to others. She is a woman who rose above abuse and lived as a survivor rather than as a victim. Ms. Winfrey turned the abuse dealt out by one man into an inspiration that has helped millions of women. Pretty impressive reframe.

One Last Word on the Echoes

Although I have spent a lot of time talking about being harmed by others in the distant past, by the time we reach adulthood most of us have committed our own fair share of transgressions against others. Being down on yourself for past mistakes or harm keeps you in the shadow lands as well. But, just like negatively ruminating on the harm by others keeps that harm alive, ruminating on our own wrongdoings is equally harmful.

In many ways I think it is harder for us, as women, to reframe our own misdeeds. But you have to if you are going to move forward in life. For lack of a better word, you have to forgive yourself in order to move forward with success. This means finding a positive meaning from a past mistake, no matter how bad it was—whether you cheated in your marriage, failed to protect a child from abuse, or even abused a child. Just like with harm done by others, finding this positive meaning depends on you and you alone. It doesn't require a ritual or asking someone to forgive you. You can if you want to. But forgiving yourself and finding a positive reframe depends on you and only you. It's a decision.

Go back to our chart and write out the five events or experiences that you most regret and the meaning you have carried with them. Now the hardest part: What can you learn from them? What kind of positive reframe can you apply to each experience? How can you turn them into something meaningful in a positive way? Much, much harder, isn't it?

If you can't value yourself enough to receive your own forgiveness, it's time to reach out. Reach out spiritually, therapeutically, or to a friend. Holding on to guilt and hurting yourself over it is just continuation of harm.

I thought this was about health and wellness. Where in this world is all this going?

I've spent a lot of time here on issues that, on the surface, seem to have little to do with health and wellness. On the contrary, it is these very deeply seated negative thinking patterns and beliefs that undermine plans for change, whether it be diet, nutrition, and exercise, or other meaningful endeavors. You have to have the fundamentals in place—optimistic language and a positive world view—to change your life for the better. If you are not taking care of yourself, if you are grossly overweight or not seeing your physician for regular check-ups, it's not because you don't know better. Most of us know what we "should" do. If you don't make healthy choices, then being down on yourself and approaching life from a negative perspective are likely getting in your way. Bitterness and pessimism are deeply rooted and deadly harmful. A health and wellness program from a personal trainer is only part of the equation—following through with the plan is the real stumbling block for most people.

Plain and simple, language and beliefs are choices that will give you either a good life or a bad one. Letting go of bitterness and pessimism is a choice. Spiritually, I am talking about accepting grace and forgiveness. Psychologically, I am talking about accepting grace and forgiveness. Socially, I am talking about accepting grace and forgiveness. You are in control of your own mind and inner life. Give yourself a chance.

Your Optimism Meter: The Present

Take stock of your world view and your language about your work, friends, and family. If you evaluated your language and world view on a continuum of optimism or pessimism, where would it fall? This goes back to the life satisfaction test you took in Chapter 2. If you are "slightly satisfied" with life, is that good enough? I hope not. When you examined the echoes from your past and your internal language and beliefs, were they more on the lighter side of the force? If so, then you are well equipped to keep on improving your life, to keep raising your game. If not, then allow me to express my concerns.

Some people get so pulled down in the negative spiral that they reach a point where they can't imagine life any other way. When I talked about not being able to reframe negative events in a winning way, this is what I meant: Hopelessness. Being in this frame of mind means you have lost hope. Without hope, you can't change anything. The hopeless person is the ultimate pessimist. When a woman lives deeply in these shadows, she desperately needs help from friends, family, and professionals. If you are this woman, reach out. If someone you love is suffering from this kind of debilitating depression, grab on to her. She needs you.

Women, being relational creatures, have the greatest source of healing right at our fingertips. We have each other. If you falter in your optimism, a clear-minded friend can help you get back on track. If you have a sister who is sinking into a negative spiral, you throw her a life preserver of hope. Depression has become a serious problem, afflicting millions of American women. It doesn't have to be this way. We devoted an entire chapter in this book to overcoming depression, but from reading this chapter you already know that the strongest weapons against living in the shadows are your language and beliefs.

Making the Change: A New Road Map

It's important to remember that when I am talking about changing your approach to life, I am talking about the mind-language *connection*—not just one or the other. Saying to yourself, "I am going to make positive affirmations my mantra" just doesn't cut it. Positive self-talk is only half of the solution. You also need to decide to be positive in your outlook.

In the beginning, your decision to be positive and your language might be a little shaky. Mine still is at times. But if you stick with it, it will take hold. Fake it till you make it. The more dedicated you become to *being* positive as well as *talking* positively, the stronger your feedback loop will become. Soon you'll be riding the wave rather than fighting to keep from drowning.

When does your commitment to optimism really matter most? When the chips are down; when you are sideswiped by life. This means giving up your allegiance to fear, worry, and other similar destructive emotions. You must embrace hope, contentment, happiness, fulfillment, satisfaction, optimism, and joy. If you will only look, you will find them every day.

There actually is a technical social science term that describes this cognitive road map: "explanatory style." This term was coined by Dr. Marty Seligman, a psychologist who revolutionized our understanding of depression, its causes, and its cures. According to Dr. Seligman, people have customary ways of explaining events, and as you now already know, these habits can be generally described as either optimistic or pessimistic.

As you may have suspected from my own life, I learned to practice optimistic principles by happenstance when I was very young. Early on in my graduate training, I did a year's stint with terminally ill children at a local hospital. Though I was a starving student, the mere exercise of going to the hospital brought me to my knees every night in thankfulness for the good people and opportunities in my life. I already had a tendency to be optimistic, but this internship really put me to the test. When I would hear a friend complain or be tempted to whine myself about some minor problem, the visualization of a frail, dying preschooler set me back on the right path. How could I complain about anything? I was alive and well, with my whole life ahead of me. I reached a point where I felt it was disrespectful to whine about anything. Though working with these sweet children was a heart-wrenching experience, I am forever thankful for their gifts to me. They taught me to live.

While I was stumbling along this road of optimism in graduate school in the 1980s, I ran across Dr. Seligman's research that I talked about earlier. There was actually social science research to support optimism as an effective weapon against depression, hopelessness, apathy, and the host of physical problems and aliments that are their comrades. I thought I had found gold, and (as it turns out) I had!

Sisters Aging with Grace

I want to share a remarkable research project on aging conducted in the United States by epidemiologist Dr. David Snowdon.[1] Much like Dr. Seligman's unexpected discoveries regarding optimism and its connection to health and wellness when he was studying depression, Dr. Snowdon, in studying aging, found his way to the very same conclusions.

Nearly twenty years ago, Dr. Snowdon, along with others, began researching aging and disease in the lives of a group of retired nuns. He reasoned that this group would be similar in terms of life experiences, since they had not been married, they had access to good medical care, they lived similar lives in terms of routines and experiences, and they were similar in social economic status (vows of poverty!) and therefore might provide some unique insight into differences in aging, health, and wellness. He affectionately called his research the Nun Study. What is absolutely remarkable about this research, though, was that the group of women who agreed to participate in this longitudinal study (research conducted over a period of years) also agreed to undergo extensive cognitive testing and mental evaluations every year, make their medical and personal histories available, and then, after death, donate their brains to the project for even further analysis. Pretty good group of girls, if you ask me.

These women gave Dr. Snowdon and his colleagues a broader and more in-depth perspective on aging and cognitive functioning than any other similar research project. These women were heroines in the truest sense.

In the course of this study, the researchers discovered that these nuns had written sketches of their lives as young novitiates in response to a request by the convent in the 1930s before taking their final vows. The autobiographies were limited to three hundred words, only one sheet of paper. The researchers examined these 180 one-page life sketches in light of the other data collected, and the findings were astonishing.

The researchers categorized the autobiographies into four groups based solely on the number of positive-emotion sentences. They were blind as to the medical history and mental functioning of who wrote which sketch. In the group with the lowest number of positive-emotion sentences, the average age of death was 86.6 years. For the next group, it was 86.8 years, then 90.0 years for the third group. For the group with the highest number of positive-emotion sentences, the life expectancy was 93.5 years. Doesn't this just rock you back on your heels? In other words, the lowest group (the lowest number of positive-emotion sentences) had twice the death risk of those in the highest group. It was clear to the researchers that a positive outlook contributed significantly to longevity. Dr. Snowdon commented that he and his colleagues actually found research support for the proverb "A merry heart doeth good like a medicine." But there's more. It turns out that the quality of life was better, too—less disease and greater resistance to cognitive decline.

Not only does optimism arm you to live life more enjoyably and effectively, it helps keep disease and illness at bay. It may be the best stress buster out there, and a good attitude is absolutely free. It's yours for the taking. Stress and depression definitely impact your quality of life, emotionally as well as physically. There is absolutely no doubt that chronic stress has long-reaching, negative health consequences. Going back to those charts of past painful events and negative interpretations, living with the negative fallout is like reliving the harm over and over; i.e., living under chronic stress. Now you have an even fuller understanding of how harmful stress can be.

Several other factors from the Nun Study are worth mentioning. Dr. Snowdon told a wonderful story about Sister Nicolette, who was the longest-surviving sister of a group of novitiates who took their vows in 1925. She survived all her classmates. When asked about her secret to long life, she cheerfully told the good doctor about her exercise program of walking several miles a day—which she started at age seventy!

Dr. Snowdon noted that she was absolutely on target with her conclusion, considering that heart disease and stroke had been the deadliest threats to this group of sisters. Good cardiac health not only fights cardiac disease and strokes (the number-one killer of women), but it improves circulation to the brain and the body. His findings fit in neatly with everything else we know about living a heart-healthy life: there are a lot of fringe benefits. Heart health means better circulation, lower blood pressure, and greater oxygen uptake to the body and brain. Avoiding vascular disease improves your chances of holding dementia or Alzheimer's disease at bay.

Women as Caregivers

We are caregivers, plain and simple. It's something we should be proud of, not apologize for. It makes the world a much better place. Since this book is by women, for women, I want to share another women's study with you that involved mothers who cared for their terminally ill children.

Researchers compared chromosome degeneration of mothers who cared for terminally ill children to mothers caring for healthy children (a non-stressed control group).[2] The caps at the end of the chromosomes in the mothers of the ill children were shortened. The length of time and the perception of the amount of stress they were under were correlated with shortened caps. Shortened caps is a condition associated with premature aging.

There were other telltale signs of premature aging of the mothers of ill children as well. Their white blood cell counts looked like those of women ten to twenty years their senior.

Hundreds upon thousands of studies show strong links between chronic stress and vulnerability to heart disease, stroke, and weakened immune systems. I could list many more but you get the picture. The bottom line? Chronic stress is bad—*very bad*.

We not only care for our children; we also care for our partners and our parents, and usually our partner's parents and the stray dog that finds its way to our house, and on and on. The U.S. Department of Health and Human Services estimated that more than fifty million people in our country provide care for a chronically ill, disabled, or aged family member or friend during any given year,[3] and that the typical family caregiver is a forty-six-year-old woman caring for a widowed mother.[4] And it looks like men are now helping out more than ever (thank goodness), as approximately 40 percent of the caretakers are men.

Many of these circumstances are joyful. Giving back is good for the heart and soul. But many of these circumstances are also chronic stress traps. So, after reading this study about these loving mothers caring for their terminally ill children, I asked myself: what real practical use does a study like this have? Plenty. It's all about how you choose to look at life, your explanatory style, and how you take care of yourself in the process.

The second half of the proverb, "A merry heart doeth good like a medicine" is "but a broken spirit drieth the bones." If you are caretaking, are you doing it with love and contentment or with anger and resentment? If it's the latter, then it's a lose-lose situation. Unless you are living in a war zone of stress that you cannot resolve or control, and some women are, you can find a way to mitigate its harmful effects. What if the mothers of the terminally ill children study had been in a support group? What if they had others helping them find joy for themselves and their child in every day? What if there were others encouraging them to exercise, eat well, stretch, meditate? Maybe, just maybe, they would be able to give care without giving out.

OPTIMISM'S MAIN INGREDIENT: Reclaiming Hope

Reaching out to others, helping others, can be gift that goes both ways.

Why did I go to the trouble to put this caregiving study at the close of this chapter? Because I know how women sometimes think. We give care to others a lot faster than we will give care to ourselves. A woman will turn her life upside down to take care of a sick partner or child, but many of us won't take an hour a day to take care of ourselves, whether it be exercising, eating a balanced meal, or meditating. If you are approaching life positively and giving to others, part of that journey will necessarily include taking care of yourself. You have to fill your own lamp first if you plan to light the way for others.

Back to the Road Map: Happiness, Health, Longevity

Happiness. Health. Longevity. By now, you know that the latter two depend on the first. Pessimism, negativity, and chronic stress lead to unhappiness, poor life satisfaction, and illness. We want you to have a terrific life, and we offer you, through the various chapters of this book, the basics that you need to get it going in the right direction. If you have had a history of failing to make the changes you want in life, things can now be different. Decide to have a better life. Make a commitment to an optimistic lifestyle. Look forward, not back. Take small steps, but keep walking. Join us and walk shoulder to shoulder with us on a new road.

PART TWO

A MOVING EXPERIENCE

Thoughts from Mary Jo:

When I was a kid, we played a game called Kick the Can. All the kids in the neighborhood gathered around a can and someone was "it." We usually had a race to determine who was going to be "it" first. We all ran and hid while the person who was "it" went to find us.

Kick the Can was much like Hide-and-Seek, except that if someone kicked the can while "it" was out looking for us, then those who had been found would be freed and we all went and hid again.

We played long past the time the sun went down. You could hear the mothers all over the neighborhood go to their back doors and call for their children. The game came to an end only when the last of us was dragged in to dinner.

We were in constant movement in those days, except when we were safely in our hiding places. None of us called it exercise; it was just fun. I remember I would go to sleep at night as soon as my head hit the pillow, and then get up the next day ready for another game of Kick the Can or Red Rover or Dodgeball.

One of the most important ingredients to a happy, healthy life is movement. As adults, unfortunately, we have classified it as "exercise" and made it yet another task on our to-do list. Our challenge is to move again, and to do it because it is fun and not because it is something we have to do.

Part 2 is not only about why movement is so important (and it is), but how we can again find joy in it.

CHAPTER 4

WITH THE WIND IN YOUR HAIR: What Aerobics Is All About

Thoughts from Mary Jo:

Running has always come easy for me. It's not that I am particularly good at it, but I like it. The inner competition I have with myself about it is very strong. Some would say that it is so strong that it renders me stupid. As a child, while in a backward-running race, I fell and fractured my arm, but I got up and won the race. As an adult, while on a ten-mile jog with two lawyers in my firm, I fell and dislocated my shoulder and fractured an elbow. We were at least five miles from the car, so in my mind the only logical thing to do was to complete the run.

Of course, I realize now that running is not supposed to be a contact sport. Even in the office, dressed in heels, if I am in a hurry I would rather break into a run than walk briskly. If I have a problem that seems insurmountable, I can go for a run and it doesn't seem as bad afterward. I am able to think it through logically and come up with an action plan. It also serves as a great stress reliever for me. Something about the rhythm of my breathing allows me to meditate, and it is often the best time I have for a conversation with God.

I am told (and have come to the conclusion that it is true) that I am just an odd duck on this issue. In fact, when I talk to Lu about running, I see the sneer that comes across her face. In fact, I think it is safe to say that she absolutely loathes it!

But, as Lu will explain, whether you run, walk, rollerblade, or ride a bike, aerobic activity is key to a healthy heart. I know that it also helps one have a positive attitude about life in general, and is helpful in preventing many cancers. There have been multiple studies that show that aerobic exercise releases neurochemicals, which then produce "feelings of elation, inner harmony, and peacefulness." [5]

When that alarm goes off at five thirty a.m. and you are nice and warm in your bed, it's hard to get up and go exercise. Or you've had a long day at work or with the kids, and you just can't see yourself going for that bike ride. I would suggest that you make a commitment to yourself that you will do something aerobic every day for a month. Write down how you felt before and after the workout, and I bet you'll see a pattern emerge—you invariably feel better afterward! Soon you won't think of exercise as drudgery, but rather as a great avenue to a "healthy high." You just may find out that you like it.

What the Exercise Physiologist Has to Say: Lu Jurcova Phillips, M.S.

Moving Forward

Our bodies are built to move. The first steps we take as toddlers are just the beginning of a lifetime of movement. As children, we move more out of pure joy—whether it's running or biking or swimming—than with any goal in mind. And that's what we want you to get back to: joy-centered movement.

I want to remind you of one of the central themes of this book. It's what you do today that matters, not what happened during the twenty or fifty years before you picked up this book. Granted, if you've been more or less inert for most of your life, you aren't going to be running a marathon in a week. But if you can get up off the couch, you will find that the joy you get from movement is worth whatever you had to do to make it happen.

The increased energy, the endorphins, the sheer joy of exerting yourself and knowing that you're giving your body what it needs—all these things will keep you coming back for more.

Benefits

Cardiovascular exercise is generally any activity that increases your workload to a level beneficial to your heart. Along with a healthy diet, cardio is, quite literally, the prescription for lifetime wellness.

Name a disease—whether it's diabetes, heart disease, Alzheimer's, cancer, fibromyalgia, obesity, or depression, to name just a few—and I can find at least one peer-reviewed medical study that links regular exercise to a reduced incidence of that disease, and a higher rate of that ailment among people who don't exercise regularly.

In other words, people who move are healthier than people who don't. They age more slowly, they're mentally sharper and less prone to accidents once they reach old age, they have better sex lives, and they get to spend their retirement years traveling through Italy as opposed to withering away in a hospital bed.

If you prefer a stiff hospital bed to Venice, then by all means, stay on the couch. For the rest of you, I'll see you on the gondolas.

Caroline: A Runner Is Born

One of my clients, a forty-seven-year-old woman we'll call Caroline, came to me complaining of low energy. She wasn't sleeping well, either. Caroline wasn't much of an exerciser—she had been an avid tennis player at one time, but hadn't done much beyond that.

Caroline was also facing osteopenia, the precursor to osteoporosis. I told her that, with some effort on her part, we could slow and possibly reverse the disease.

After assessing her, I decided she should try running. Now, running isn't for everyone, and having proper form is important to prevent injuries. But fortunately Caroline was working with a personal trainer who could address incorrect form before it became a problem.

We started out with ten minutes of jogging, three times a week, as a warm-up to doing her strength-training workout. She later added a thirty- to forty-five-minute walk twice a week. We gradually worked her up to fifteen minutes and then thirty minutes of jogging.

Caroline decided she wanted to try a 5K (which she conquered), and she began shooting for a 10K—and then she was hooked. Since then, she's been running in a race just about every month. She's also had increased energy levels and has been sleeping much better. Best of all, her osteopenia has reversed.

WITH THE WIND IN YOUR HAIR: What Aerobics Is All About

Scott: From Biker to *Biker*

One of my favorite clients is Scott, a fifty-something lawyer who, on his weekends, liked to ride motorcycles. Unfortunately, sitting in that unnatural position for so long caused him hip pain.

I advised him to try some spin classes to strengthen and tone his tortured hip flexors. It's almost the same position as he was sitting in on his motorcycle, but it added the element of movement. We also worked on strength training to take the pressure off his hip flexors, which were overloaded, causing those muscles to knot up and tighten.

Scott loved the spin class so much that he started riding in the "real world" on an old mountain bike. He quickly moved up to a lighter, faster road bike and started tackling longer rides. He's become such an avid cyclist that, for the last three years, Scott has ridden in an annual 150-mile weekend ride.

He still enjoys his motorcycle, but the "real" biking keeps him in shape to handle the stress of his weekday *and* his weekend life.

Now a Little Science

Cardiovascular/cardiorespiratory fitness allows a person to sustain an activity for a prolonged period of time. It allows the lungs to provide oxygen to the blood and, in turn, for the heart to deliver the oxygenated blood to the cells of the body, including muscles. Along with oxygen, blood also delivers nutrients to body parts that need them.

Good blood circulation allows for proper movement of our arms and legs, and also for adequate brain functioning. Poor circulation is demonstrated by several symptoms, such as neuropathy (tingling or loss of sensation in the hands and feet), shortness of breath, a lack of energy, irregular heartbeat, and impaired memory. Some of the conditions linked to poor circulation are

A Happy Healthy You

arthritis, angina, high blood pressure, heart disease, diabetes, and high LDL (bad) cholesterol.

The better your cardiorespiratory fitness, the more blood you deliver with each beat of your heart. This means your heart doesn't have to work as hard to circulate blood around your body. Your heart acts as an engine in your body, and the less work it has to do to pump the blood in your system, the less fatigued it gets. A fit person has a much younger heart than a person who spends most of her time channel surfing on her couch. Do not confuse channel surfing with a sport.

Cardiorespiratory fitness means:

1. An increase in cardiac output (the total amount of blood pumped by the ventricle in one minute)
2. An increase in lung capacity, giving you greater stamina
3. An increase in calorie-burning ability
4. An increase in metabolic rate
5. An increase in HDL (good) cholesterol
6. A decrease in body fat
7. A decrease in total cholesterol
8. A decreased risk for diabetes

Of course, medical benefits that you may not see until your sixties or seventies may be compelling, but you're looking for short-term benefits, right? How about these:

1. Increased energy
2. Better, deeper, more restful sleep
3. Better moods
4. Stress relief
5. Increased mental capacity and ability to focus

These are all benefits you can experience this week after just a few good workouts. So, now that I've convinced you of the benefits of regular exercise, what's next?

Put One Foot in Front of the Other

If you don't already have an exercise regimen, the best way to get started is to put one foot in front of the other—literally. Walking is and has always been the most popular form of exercise on earth. It's restful, you don't need any special equipment (except good shoes) or skills, it's easy, and you can do it on your own schedule. You can also buy or rent walking DVDs that you can do in your living room (without a treadmill), so you don't even have to leave your house.

Walking can be as relaxing or as rigorous as your body can handle. Just getting started? Try ten minutes at a slow pace, and build on that as you get more fit. If you're already in decent shape, start with thirty to sixty minutes at a brisk pace.

Eventually, and ideally, you'll be doing cardio for an hour a day, seven days a week. It doesn't have to be a solid sixty minutes, either. You can do three twenty-minute sessions, two thirty-minute sessions—however you want to break it up to make it fit with your schedule. One of my clients runs in the morning and uses her evening walk as a relaxing end to her hectic schedule. At this point, she could do her entire workout in one session, but she found a more enjoyable way to do it, and this helps her stick to it.

Intensity

If you're just getting started, don't worry about intensity yet. If 90 percent of success means showing up, then just getting out of bed, getting dressed, and heading out the door is victory.

Low intensity is fine to start with, but we don't want to stay there forever. Sooner rather than later, you'll want to kick it up a notch. If the walk you've been doing isn't challenging you, pick it up a bit. Our muscles have a keen ability to adapt to what we demand of them. If they no longer seem to be working hard to finish a thirty-minute walk at three miles per hour, go longer or walk faster. As long as you're out there, you may as well work hard.

How do you know if you're working hard enough? Your heart rate will tell you. Now it's time for the math portion of the program.

Let's say you're forty years old. To calculate your estimated maximum heart rate, subtract your age from 220. So, 220 - 40 (your age) = 180 beats per minute (bpm). That's your maximum heart rate.

Now, to calculate your targeted heart rate zone, multiply your maximum heart rate by the desired percentage. Low intensity exercise—one that beginners are able to sustain for a prolonged period of time—is 65 percent of your maximum heart rate. So, if you're forty, your target for low-intensity exercise is 117 bpm, or 180 x 0.65. At this intensity level, your body is burning mostly fat. As your body gets used to the demands of a low-intensity workload, however, it's time to do more.

Once you increase the intensity, you're burning both fat and glucose. Burning glucose is important, because it prevents the body from storing more fat. When glucose consumption exceeds the body's energy needs, it is broken down into smaller particles, diverted from the energy production pathways, and starts building fat for energy storage. You'll want to stay in the 65 percent to 85 percent range of your maximum heart rate. Our forty-year-old example would want to shoot for between 117 and 153 bpm.

Why not shoot higher than 85 percent for the whole workout? Because anything above 85 percent of your maximum heart rate does not qualify as aerobic activity. The demands on the energy production at that point are too high, and therefore no oxygen is used. Instead, you're burning glycogen. You may find yourself exceeding 85 percent occasionally, but you don't want to maintain that level for the duration of your workout.

One word of caution about heart rate calculations: they are, by design, quite general and don't take into account things like gender or fitness differences. We all know forty-year-olds who can climb Mt. Everest and others who get winded climbing into bed. So, the standard 220-minus-your-age calculation isn't always reliable. Unless you have gone through a maximum oxygen uptake test at a sports medicine clinic or your doctor's office, use this number as a mere estimate.

Why You Should Get a Heart Rate Monitor

The easiest way to know how hard your heart is working is to purchase a heart rate monitor (HRM). These little devices come at different price levels. Unless you plan on training for a specific race, I would not recommend spending money on the bells and whistles advanced HRMs offer. Just stick to the basics. Find a monitor that allows you to view your heart rate. I am partial to Polar heart rate monitors, while others prefer Acumen. As your training needs require more specific help, you may opt for updating your HRM. The Polar Web site, www.polarusa.com, can help buyers select the right HRM for their needs. Whether you get a basic HRM or one with lots of bells and whistles, you'll want to get one. It will make your training much more efficient.

HRMs feature a strap you wear around your chest and a receiver (worn like a wristwatch) that wirelessly receives information from the strap and calculates your heart rate. You do not have to worry about straps and connectors, just the wristwatch and chest strap. Chances are, you're already wearing a sports bra, so for us, the strap isn't bothersome.

Now, back to the unreliability issue of maximum heart rate. If you have a heart rate monitor, you will know exactly how fast your heart is beating. If you're registering 153, which if you're forty should be as high as you want to go for an extended period of time, and you're barely breaking a sweat, feel free to work harder. In time, you'll learn what you can handle and when your heart rate's going into the red zone.

You should be able to say, "Hi, how are you doing?" in one breath while exercising. If you can't, you're probably working too hard and won't be able to sustain that level. Slow down a little and try the "talk test" again in a few minutes.

One way to make your calculated target heart zones more individualized is using the Karnoven method. You take the same base number of 220, minus your age, minus your resting heart rate. This calculation gives you what we call your "heart rate reserve." To get your target heart zones, you can use the heart rate reserve to calculate the percentages and then add your resting heart rate back into the equation.

For example: a forty-year-old woman with a resting heart rate of fifty beats per minute (bpm). Heart rate reserve = 220 - 40 (age) - 50 (resting heart rate) = 130 bpm.

65 percent max = (130 bpm x 0.65) + 50 bpm = 134.5 bpm
75 percent max = (130 bpm x 0.75) + 50 bpm = 147.5 bpm
85 percent max = (130 bpm x 0.85) + 50 bpm = 160.5 bpm

As you can see, the lower your resting heart rate, the higher your target heart zones appear to be. This is not an accident. As you get in better cardiorespiratory shape, your body can withstand a more demanding workload.

How do you determine your resting heart rate? The best time to do it is early in the morning while you are still lying in bed. Ideally, you'll want to do it on the weekend or a morning when you won't have an alarm clock going off, artificially ratcheting up your heart rate. If you're wearing your heart rate monitor, you can simply use that to determine your resting heart rate. You can also check it manually by counting the number of heartbeats for one minute. To find your pulse, simply place your index finger (not your thumb) on the inside of your wrist.

Ideally, as you become more fit, your resting heart rate will decrease. If you notice an increase, lower the intensity of your workouts until it goes back down.

What Is the Best Cardio?

The great thing about movement is that there are so many different ways to do it. And every day there seem to be new sports popping up created by people who just can't get enough movement.

For most of us, though, the basics are all we need. The form of exercise you choose is limited only by your desire, your imagination, and your physical condition when you start exercising. The possibilities are endless, as long as you do something that elevates your heart rate.

I advise most of my clients to start with walking, just to get their bodies accustomed to regular movement. Most of us, though, need a little variety to keep ourselves interested, so don't be afraid to try something new.

Your local gym probably has a whole schedule of cardio classes, including spinning, trekking, kickboxing, low-impact aerobics, water aerobics, Zumba (the latest craze in dance aerobics), and many, many more. Some gyms even offer classes that incorporate weight training.

Many of my clients prefer cardio classes to anything they can do on their own, because the instructor provides motivation and, often, great music. Additionally, the camaraderie of others in your class can keep you coming back.

Lap swimming is also one of the most popular and healthful sports around, although it can be difficult to do for an extended period of time. Unless you are a trained swimmer, it may be difficult for you to swim hard enough to increase your heart rate and sustain that intensity for the duration of your workout. But don't be discouraged. Take it one day at a time and you will get there.

Gyms also offer a seemingly endless array of cardio machines. Treadmills, stationary bikes, stair climbers, arc trainers, and ellipticals are the most popular. The downside is that some people find machines too boring to do for long periods of time. If you're one of those people, use the machines only as a backup to your more favored activities.

Don't like exercising indoors? Fantastic. The great outdoors is for you. Running, hiking, biking, kayaking, and open-water swimming are great ways to commune with nature while working up a sweat. Of course, exercising outdoors poses risks that you need to be prepared for. The weather is an obvious factor, as are road hazards, pollution, injuries, etc. If you'll be exercising in a remote area, take a buddy, a cell phone, and plenty of water. If you're biking, take a tire repair kit. If you're hiking, take a map and know your bearings. You get the picture.

One other possibility is home workout DVDs or videos. Ever since Jane Fonda slipped on that first pair of leg-warmers and told us to "feel the burn," workout videos and DVDs have been selling like hotcakes. Like any other form of exercise, it may be for you, or it may not be. You just have to try it out to see if it is. Some libraries and video rental outlets have workout videos and DVDs you can rent or borrow, so feel free to try before you buy.

If you're in a rut, try something new. Feel the joy of pushing your body to the limit and coming back for more. You won't regret it.

What About Intervals?

If you have ever taken a spin class, you know what intervals are. You go at a steady pace for a few minutes, then your instructor cranks up the music and tells you to sprint for thirty seconds. More generally, intervals are longer, slower periods of exercise broken up by short, fast bursts of intensity.

Intervals are fun. They're hard. And they're a great way to increase your endurance. During the short, hard intervals, the body starts to build new capillaries, which aid in better uptake and delivery of oxygen to the working muscles. The heart muscle itself strengthens through the process, and the muscles become more tolerant to the buildup of lactate. Intervals also bring the anaerobic (non-oxygen producing) energy production system into our aerobic workout, and these fast, brief bursts of power help us strengthen bones and build muscles. Adding interval training to your routine makes it more enjoyable. It makes you less susceptible to burnout, and some experts believe it helps prevent injury, because it allows the body to perform the same movement differently. Plus, for those of you not yet a fan of exercise, if you know you're only going to be working really, really hard for thirty seconds to a minute, it makes it more tolerable.

You'll want to start slow, however. There are four main variables that play a part in your interval training:

1. The duration of the work interval
2. The duration of your recovery interval
3. The intensity of your work interval
4. The number of intervals throughout the routine

Feel free to vary these often. Allow your muscles to go through a proper warm-up at the beginning of your workout, and let your heart rate go back down to a slower rate during the recovery intervals before you increase the intensity again.

Once you've been exercising regularly for a while, you'll wonder how you ever went a day without it. Our bodies were not built to be sedentary, yet our lifestyle demands so little movement from us that we can no longer get physical activity just from our daily lives.

We cook, we gather food, we do laundry, we go from point A to point B—all with a minimum of physical exertion. Even the most undemanding of tasks—watching television—has become lazier with the proliferation of the remote control.

It's time to give your body what it craves: movement. And lots of it. Recapture the joy of your youth. Get outside. Play. Have fun. Your body will thank you for it.

I have included below a sample program of exercises for you to use or modify to your lifestyle or preferences.

Beginner's Cardio Program

At first, aim for twenty to thirty minutes, two to three times a week, with a few days of rest in between to allow your body to recover.

Start each workout with a five-minute walk for a warm-up.

If using a treadmill, have the incline on at least 1 percent to avoid getting help from the motor.

If walking:

1. Find your comfort level and walk for twenty minutes at that pace.
2. Over the next three weeks, gradually increase your speed.
3. On week 4, start raising the incline for a few minutes at a time, bringing it back down to 1 percent to allow your body to recover.

4. If you're using a treadmill, don't hold on to the bars. You should be able to use your abdominal muscles to help you balance. If you're not comfortable walking uphill without holding on, stay with the incline at 1 percent.

If running:

1. You may choose to use time or distance as units of measurement (i.e., ten minutes or 0.25 mile, etc.)
2. For the first three weeks, begin with a 1:2 ratio of jogging to walking (e.g., jog for thirty seconds, walk for sixty seconds, or jog for 0.1 mile, walk for 0.2 mile.)
3. Find your comfort zone and stick to it for three weeks to prepare your body for running without injury.
4. At week 4, you may begin to increase your time/distance of running intervals and decrease your walking interval.
5. After a few weeks, there will be no need to have walking intervals.

Injury Prevention

To prevent injuries that can sideline you completely, you need to listen to your body. If you're feeling joint pain (especially in the knees, hips, and ankles), don't just try to "work through it." Either there's a muscle imbalance that needs to be addressed or there's an injury and you're just making it worse. Stop running until the pain stops and then try again. If the injury comes back, stop again and perhaps seek medical help.

People who haven't been running sometimes have trouble with shin splints—tingly, achy pain in the front of your legs that runs the length of your shin. That's something you can work through. It's just inflammation and gets healed over time as you become more active. A good treatment is to freeze some water in a small cup and run it up and down your shin for five to seven minutes.

CHAPTER 5

CURLING IRON: Strength Training

Thoughts from Mary Jo:

I still remember the day I was in the college cafeteria and one of my "friends" started clucking like a chicken when he saw me coming across the room in my shorts. I had to face it: I had no shape in my legs, even though I ran and played tennis. I figured it would always be that way. Imagine my surprise when, at the age of thirty-nine, I was taking an aerobics class where you hold three- or five-pound weights in your hand and, after only two weeks, I began seeing some definition in my arms and legs. I was hooked, and so was my good friend Paula. We immediately sought out a strength trainer at our club. We shared the cost and hired him together to begin strength training. But what I started because of vanity turned out to be one of the best things I had ever done.

One year later, at the age of forty, I had my first bone density test. The doctor told me I had osteopenia (just short of osteoporosis). How could this be? I run and I lift weights! The doctor calmly explained that blonde, blue-eyed, small-frame women are more susceptible to osteoporosis; further, if I had not been running and lifting weights it likely would already have become osteoporosis. Actually, my hips were in normal range, probably because of the running, but my spine was dangerously close to being over the line.

The scariest part of osteoporosis is that it has no warning signs. One day you just break something, without any explanation. My vanity actually saved me, but now I had to get down to serious work. I had to pay particular attention to the muscles around my spine. Sixteen years later, I'm still working out with weights. Every year my bones have either gotten better or stayed the same. I have not crossed that invisible line into osteoporosis.

The good news is that it really isn't hard. I work out with weights two times or, at most, three times a week. While it is great if you can hire someone like Lu to get you started with proper form, if you can't, there are other options. If you belong to a gym or a YWCA, have someone spend at least two sessions with you, to show you proper form and some basic exercises. Don't feel like you have to do all the fancy moves you may see others doing. Learn five or six strength exercises that work all the major muscle groups. If you don't belong to a gym, buy or rent a video, but be sure to stick with lighter weights until you are sure your form is correct, and you won't injure yourself.

You know the commercial, "I've fallen and I can't get up?" To make sure that isn't you, read the rest of this chapter! It may save you from a lot of heart- (and hip- and back-) ache.

CURLING IRON: Strength Training

What the Exercise Physiologist Has to Say: Lu Jurcova Phillips, M.S.

For the most part, I like gravity. It literally keeps us grounded, and we'd be lost without it. But as we age, it can also be our enemy, pulling us down and putting stress on our bones. For better or worse, gravity's here to stay, so what can we do about it? The answer is strength training.

Resistance training, strength training, weight lifting, weight training—they all mean the same thing. Every time you move a dumbbell, push the arm of a Cyber machine, or pull on a cable hanging from a free-motion tower, you are working against the resistance of that particular piece of equipment. You are curling iron.

Muscles are stimulated when we require them to work. If you do consistent strength training, you can improve your coordination, balance, overall circulation, ligament and bone strength, and durability. My clients have a love/hate relationship with this kind of work. They love it because they feel so great afterward, and they hate it because—and there's no other way to put this—it can hurt.

But the pain we feel from exercise is nothing compared to the pain of aching joints. And that is exactly what we prevent when we strengthen our muscles. Muscle strength helps our joints handle their daily workload. Well-developed muscles support our bodies and prevent injury. And because strength training promotes good blood flow and circulation, the ligaments, tendons, and cartilage that help hold us together stay lubricated and healthy. Without good circulation, those critical components can dry out and crumble.

In the event of an earthquake, experts tell us to stand in a doorway because that is typically the best-constructed, sturdiest part of the house. My goal is to make sure your "doorway" is sturdy enough to endure not only the daily pressure of holding up your house, but also the occasional earthquake, such as a fall or an accident.

Another benefit of strength training is that it helps increase our metabolism. Our bodies expend energy at a rate that is defined by many factors, including our age, genetics, and activity levels. When we increase our muscle mass, we burn calories at a much higher rate. This comes in handy when you're trying to fit into a smaller pair of jeans.

A Good Workout Mimics Everyday Life

Most of the strength-training exercises you should be doing closely mimic the movements we all perform on a regular basis. We all have to squat and reach while trying to pull out that one yogurt snack pack from the bottom drawer of the refrigerator. Doing overhead presses will help you the next time you get on an airplane and have to hoist your carry-on bag into the overhead compartment. Doing push-ups may even help you push away from the table! Even if all you want is to be able to play on the floor with your dogs and get up without hurting yourself, strength training can help.

Strengthening Bones

For women, the best thing about strength training is what it does for our bones. Like any other living tissue, bones respond to exercise by becoming stronger and healthier. Two kinds of exercise accomplish this: weight-bearing activities and strength training. Weight-bearing exercise is movement of your body against gravity, and includes activities like walking, jogging, and dancing. Strength training, such as lifting weights and doing push-ups, build muscle mass.

Weight-bearing exercises and strength training help create stronger, denser bones, because our muscles are attached to our bones. When you place demands on a muscle, it contracts, pulling on the point of attachment to the bone. This stresses the bone itself, creating a stronger, denser bone. Frail bones—the kind of bones we're trying to avoid—are rarely challenged.

Two years ago, Judy, a client of mine in her late forties, was told she was on the borderline of having osteoporosis. Many people, including Judy, tend to associate osteoporosis exclusively with the frail and elderly. While it can certainly make you feel frail and old, osteoporosis is not unheard of in younger people. And Judy, an avid tennis player who takes good care of herself, certainly didn't think she would ever be at risk for it.

Although Judy was skeptical that something as simple as a workout could reverse her diagnosis, she and I mapped out a strategy and got to work. Judy's workout consisted mostly of weight-bearing exercise, primarily walking and strength training that focused on holding the weights at hip or shoulder level.

Her workout included moves such as doing squats while holding a bar on her shoulders and performing lunges while holding dumbbells at her waist. This put stress on the hips and spine and helped to strengthen those crucial structures.

Both because it's better for bone strengthening and because it more closely mimics real life, in situations like Judy's I prefer using free weights in a standing position rather than using machines or doing free weights in a seated position. And because you're using your core muscles—the muscles in your back and abdomen—to stabilize yourself, you're strengthening those as well.

After Judy and I had been working together for two years, she walked into our studio with some papers in her hand and a big smile on her face. She had just gotten the results of her latest bone mineral density test, and the results were great. Together we had reversed the progress osteoporosis had made in her body. It made my—and Judy's—day.

Judy's results aren't unique. I've seen many clients transform their bodies through strength training. They feel better, they look better, they're healthier, and they're much less likely to face osteoporosis down the road. There's no reason to wait, as Judy did, until you've received an alarming bone density scan to start weight training.

Emily: From Osteoporosis to Solid as a Rock

Emily made no bones about it when she came in to see me. She hated weight lifting and was there for only two reasons: 1) her husband, a client of mine, insisted she do it; and 2) the small matter of osteoporosis in her spine.

Emily was already quite active. She had been a swimmer and a runner and was in good shape. But her osteoporosis diagnosis frightened her and jolted her into action, albeit reluctantly. Unfortunately, the most I could get out of her was once-a-week training. Normally, I don't even bother with someone who wants to work out only once a week. It shows a lack of commitment, and you need to come in at least twice a week to see any results. But after some cajoling, I agreed to start her out with a once-a-week appointment.

I fitted Emily with a weight vest, which looks a bit like a bulletproof vest and allows you to add weight to your frame—a big plus if you're working against osteoporosis in the spine. She did squats, shoulder presses, chest flies, lunges, and step-ups. I had Emily do all her exercises standing up because that more closely mimics daily life.

Machines tend to stabilize the body and don't work any part but the specific muscle group targeted by the machine. In real life, though, as you're stooping to pick up laundry or grass clippings, or reaching for a dish at the top of your cupboard, there's nothing stabilizing you but your own muscles. So my clients will typically do their workouts while standing.

I won't say that Emily ever came to *love* working out, but she certainly loved the results. She moved up to twice- and then three-times-a-week workouts. Not only does this fifty-six-year-old now have a body any thirty-year-old would envy, but her osteoporosis has actually *reversed*.

Sara: A Benched Tennis Ace Gets to Reclaim the Sport She Loves

Sara, fifty-five, was an avid tennis player but had never gotten into weight training. However, while playing tennis, she tore her meniscus, the cartilage in her knee. Unfortunately, cartilage doesn't regenerate, and the torn meniscus simply floated around in her knee and caused her pain. Sara had to give up her favorite sport because it simply hurt too much to play. Determined not to leave tennis behind forever, she started working out with me.

Sara needed to strengthen her leg muscles, which we accomplished by doing lots of lunges and doing her strength-training routine while standing on one leg and/or seated on a Bosu ball (a dome-shaped piece of equipment you've probably seen at the gym). We also worked on Sara's core muscles, which provide stability for the entire body.

By strengthening the muscles around her knees (and throughout her body), Sara was able to take the pressure off the area of her injury. After a few months of regular workouts, Sara was back on the courts and playing the sport she loves.

A Word about Soreness and "Bulking Up"

Many women are reluctant to start strength training because they are worried about being sore. They shouldn't be. Soreness is a normal response to unusual exertion, and is part of the adaptation process that leads to greater stamina and strength as the muscles recover and rebuild. The first two days are often the worst, but the pain typically subsides over the next few days.

Soreness is caused by microscopic tears in muscle fibers often followed by localized swelling. The amount of tearing and the resulting soreness depends greatly on the types of exercises you do. Contrary to popular belief, the soreness is not caused by the formation of waste products in muscles, such as lactic acid. Because lactic acid disperses fairly rapidly, it would not explain soreness after several hours or days. Ironically, some women who don't want to start strength training because of the soreness actually come to enjoy it, almost as a badge of courage. Regardless, the soreness becomes less severe as your muscles become more fit.

Another fear many women have about strength training is that it will make them bigger—a goal few ladies care to pursue. Fortunately, this is an unfounded fear. Unless a woman is taking steroids (which I can't recommend against strongly enough), she will never get huge muscles, simply because the average woman has twenty to thirty times less testosterone than men do.

Through strength training, we develop sleek, defined muscles that help us burn calories more efficiently. We can all agree that's a positive goal.

Core Strength

Core strength is all the rage these days. Most gyms offer multiple core-strengthening classes, and it's impossible to turn on the TV or go into a bookstore or fitness store without seeing core workout books, DVDs, and stability balls.

The "core" encompasses the muscles of the abdomen and back. It consists of all the tiny, deep muscles that attach to the spine or the pelvis, and we use them as a stability platform. The abs and back work together to support our spine as we do everything from standing in line to catching ourselves in a fall.

Without core strength, we are unable to achieve maximum strength in any other muscle in our bodies. The core works as a center of stabilizing power, which is why it's called "the powerhouse."

As you begin your strength-training journey, do not neglect your core. Strengthening your "powerhouse" is not just a fun addition to your workout. It is absolutely critical.

How to Start When You Just Don't Feel Like It

Many of us believe that we must have everything completely under control before we attempt to start something new. We say things like, "I'll get to the gym once I get the kitchen redone," or "as soon as we get past the third quarter," or "once the kids are back in school." Trust me, there will never be a time when your life is completely under control and you suddenly find yourself with an extra hour a day to devote to your health. Like everything else that matters, you simply must find the time and make it happen.

You don't need to do everything all at once. Plan to spend your first few weeks learning the ropes, trying out different exercises, and determining which ones you and your body like best. With time, you can build up to a full routine that will get you in peak shape.

Go ahead: pack your gym bag and head to the gym. Sign up for an introductory session with a trainer. Many gyms offer complimentary "getting started" sessions for new members. Let an expert show you how to use the machines and free weights. Take note of which muscles each exercise targets. When you're working out, think—literally—about the muscle you're supposed to be working. You will have a more intense workout.

Start slowly. If you're new to strength training, use lighter weights with more repetitions. Let your body get used to this new level of exertion. You may be using muscles you didn't even know existed.

Don't overdo it. If you have trouble getting out of your car or climbing the handful of steps into your office building, you may want to scale your workout back a bit. Of course you will experience some soreness, but it shouldn't be extremely painful or cause limitations in your daily activities. Remember, curling iron is supposed to improve your quality of life, not cripple you.

Warm Up Before and Stretch After

A proper warm-up routine is key to preventing injuries. I recommend doing ten minutes on the stationary bike or treadmill to increase the blood flow in your muscles, followed by doing an "unloaded" version of the exercise you'll be doing, or using very light weights. It's important to get blood flowing into the muscles you'll be working, because if your muscles aren't warm, they won't have the energy to do the work you're asking of them, and your joints will take over to do the job. That's when injuries can happen.

At the end of your workout, it's important to do some brief stretching, which will help reduce soreness and post-workout muscle tightening. While stretching, it's important to listen to your body and not force it where it doesn't want to go. A muscle should be stretched only to the point where you feel a good stretch but no pain. You don't want a stretch to feel as if your muscles are going to tear apart. Hold that stretch for ten to twenty seconds without pain. Continue breathing properly throughout the stretch. Many people stop breathing when they're focused on something, but that can work against you by depriving your muscles of the oxygen they need to perform. Focus on deep breathing, and see if you can deepen your stretch on the exhalation. The carbon dioxide coming out of your bloodstream allows you to relax.

Picking a Trainer

If you hire a trainer, even if it's only for a few sessions, be choosy. Ask about her education and whether she has any additional certifications. Look for nationally recognized certifications, such as the

National Academy of Sports Medicine (NASM) and the National Strength and Conditioning Association (NSCA). Be skeptical if the only certification the trainer has is from the gym that signs her paycheck. Also look for continuing education—a sign that she's up on the latest research and technology.

Make sure your trainer does a full-body assessment, looking for your strengths and weaknesses. Without one, it will be very difficult for her to write up an individualized program. Finally, get to know your trainer. She will be your guide on your new adventure. Let her help you.

If you work out without a trainer, allow yourself a session or two every six weeks. That way, she can tweak your program and make changes depending on your progress. Why tweak your workout program? Because our bodies adapt to the demands we put on them. After six weeks or so of the same workout, our bodies don't feel challenged anymore, and you want to keep your body guessing. By changing your workout periodically, you'll see faster, better results.

With that said, be patient. Major changes take time. Develop a workout plan you can live with. If you vow to work out two hours a day, six days a week, you're probably setting yourself up for failure. But if you shoot for two to three times a week for an hour or so each time, that's a plan you can probably live with.

It took you a lifetime to develop the habits—and the body—you have now. It will take time to develop new habits and a new body.

When Is the Best Time to Work Out?

The best time to work out is whenever you will do it. Your neighbor or best friend may prefer going to the gym at night, but just because it works for her doesn't mean it will work for you. Each of us has different body rhythms and different energy levels. You probably already know what yours are. Don't work against them.

For most women, the best time to work out is early in the morning or later in the evening. This is for one very practical reason: we don't want to have to shower, wash our hair, and do our makeup more than once a day.

It may take you a few weeks to figure out your optimal time to work out. Once you do, though, make it a priority. Put it on your calendar and don't schedule other things during that time, even if you promise yourself you'll get to the gym another time during the day. You won't.

Plan ahead. Have your bag packed and ready to go. Mine has all the necessary items: my iPod, shower flip-flops, workout clothes (preferably a matching outfit, because I like to look good), shoes, and socks. I find that if you have to locate everything at the last minute, it's too easy to throw in the towel and skip the gym that day. Keep in mind many gyms today provide you with towels, shampoo, conditioner, soap, lotion, and deodorant. But make yourself a checklist on an index card. Include clothes, shoes, toiletries, MP3 player—everything you need to get your workout in—and keep these in your bag. Nothing is worse than getting to the gym and realizing you've left your underwear at home.

Companionship as a Motivator

Having a workout buddy also helps. For women, companionship may be the single most important motivator to exercise. Women are social creatures. We've been bonding and gossiping over coffee and lunch since the dawn of time. Now we can bond during workouts. Ask your girlfriend, co-worker, daughter, mother, sister—even your husband or boyfriend—to work out with you. Make a date and stick to it. The prospect of visiting with a friend may be just the incentive you need to get yourself to the gym after a long day at the office.

If you don't have any friends outside the gym who will go with you, look around the gym. After a few weeks, you'll probably see some of the same faces there at the same time you are. Consider asking one of your gym mates to be a workout buddy. Remember, they're there for the same reason you are: to get in shape.

I'll grant you, there will be times you don't want to go to the gym. At first, it may be every time. But there will come a day when you will honestly look forward to your workout and can't go a day without it. That day will be your greatest reward.

Music as a Motivator

Maybe you don't have a workout buddy or you only get together once a week. What's the best way to get going? Music. I urge my clients to have a variety of different music on their MP3 players. They may want something moderately peppy for their warm-up, hard-charging for the meat of their workout, and fairly mellow for their cool down. And different days may mean different moods.

One of my clients uses Tina Turner or Elton John every time she needs a slight kick to get herself going. Recently her twenty-year-old son bought her an iPod, and she now has a wider variety to choose from. I suspect she still turns to Tina and Elton, though, when she needs that extra push.

Curling Iron: Three Times a Week

I recommend doing weight training three times a week. Give yourself a day of rest between workouts so that your muscles can recover. Recovery is key to improvement. When you lift weights, you develop little tears in your muscle fibers, and the recovery time allows them to rebuild and grow stronger.

Stick to full-body workouts. That way, each muscle group gets challenged each of the three times a week you come in. Eventually you may want a more challenging workout and need to break down your workouts into upper- and lower-body days, front- and back-muscle days, etc. But when you do that, your number of visits needs to increase.

It helps to have a goal. If you do, share that with your trainer so she can help you get there. It can be a vacation at a national park with tons of hiking, a dress you've been dying to wear, or avoiding a condition that runs in your family. These are just a few of what I call "initial motivators."

Once you've made progress toward—or even achieved—your initial goal (see chapter 16) you may want to set another one. You would be surprised how often that happens. You may begin strength training to help your back pain, but in the process, you get sucked into a group that's training for a hiking trip in six months. There's a new goal! If you change your goal, consult your trainer again and let her assess your progress and modify your program accordingly. It's like taking a road trip with an updated map. You want to make sure that all the newly developed roads are included.

Regardless of what made you start working out in the first place, once you get into a regular workout routine, you will realize that the number-one motivator, the one that will last for as long as you need it to pull from, is your health. If you keep at your program, your health will improve. You'll feel better, you'll have more energy, and you'll sleep better. The dress you were trying so hard to fit into may go out of style, but great health never does.

Choosing a Gym

For many women, gyms are scary places. We picture the dank, smelly gyms in movies like *Rocky*, and there are all sorts of intimidating, confusing pieces of equipment that look more like implements of torture than tools of beautification.

Don't be intimidated. First off, most gyms these days are sunny and welcoming, even to the most novice exercisers. And after a few weeks of workouts, those "torture tools" will be your best friends.

First and foremost, find a gym that's close to you, either on your way to and from work, or near your house or office. Don't let geography stand between you and your workout.

The fitness industry offers an array of choices. The large chains can be a bit overwhelming at first. It's easy to get lost and feel like "one of the pack." On the other hand, some people prefer that level of anonymity, particularly if they spend all day in front of people. Smaller studios also have their advantages. They're more intimate, and I have found that people who go to smaller gyms tend to be more focused on their workout. They also tend to be more regular and attend on the same days, at the same time. Because of this, the people who frequent these gyms can become tight-knit.

In either environment, on a tough day you'll find that the positive atmosphere in the gym and all the active people around you can motivate you more than you expected. Use that to your advantage and feed off it whenever you can.

Your Goals, Not Your Neighbor's

One thing to remember: focus only on your progress toward your goals. Don't compare yourself to others, whether it's your neighbor, best friend, or whichever starlet graced the cover of last month's *Vogue*. We are all different, with different genes, health issues, body types, and energy levels. Two women can do the same workout program and have different results. It's not fair, but it's true. Don't let that discourage you. The changes you are making now will make you a healthier, happier woman, able to face even the most daunting challenges life throws at you.

I have included a few examples of a basic strength-training workout below.

A Happy Healthy You

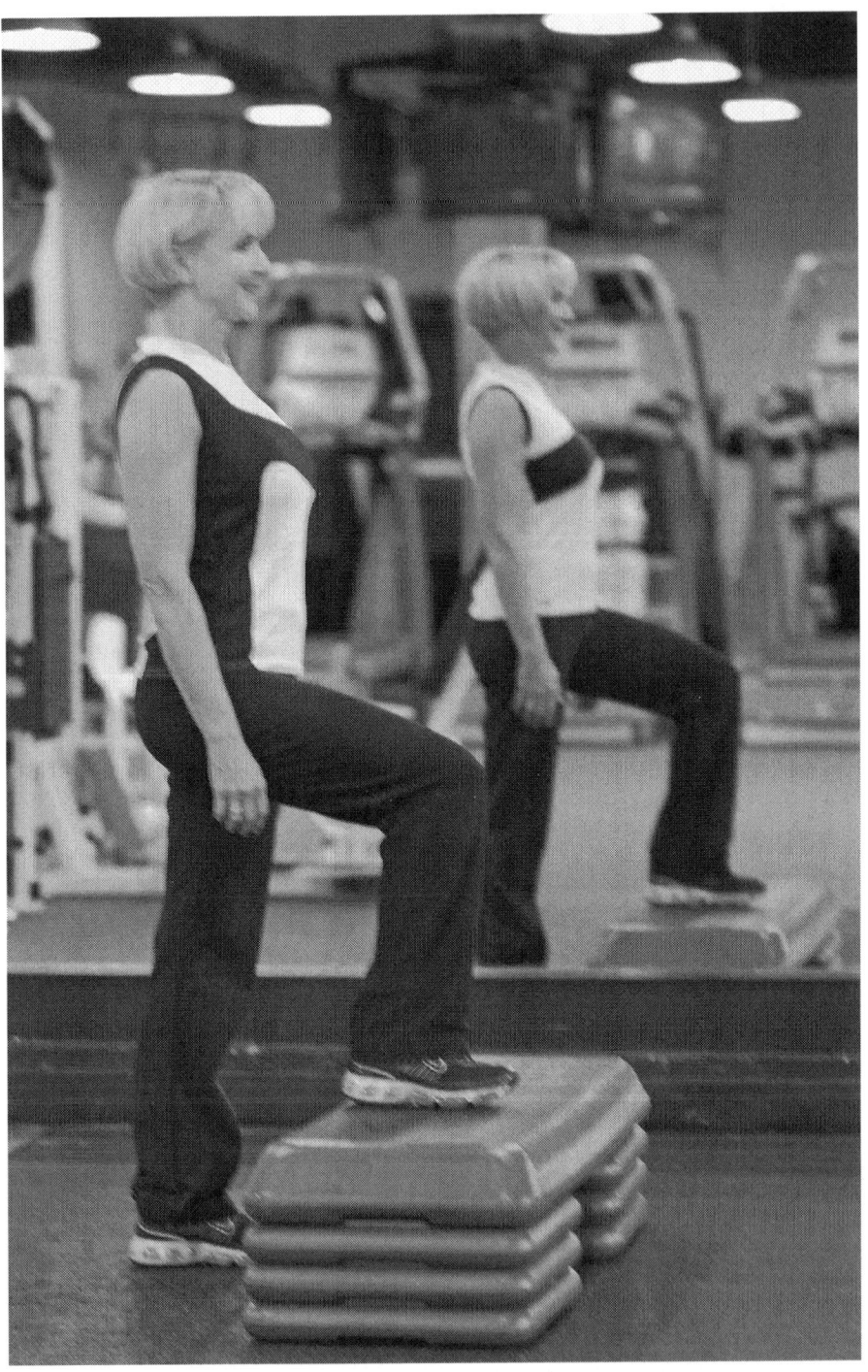

Bench Step-up – Start

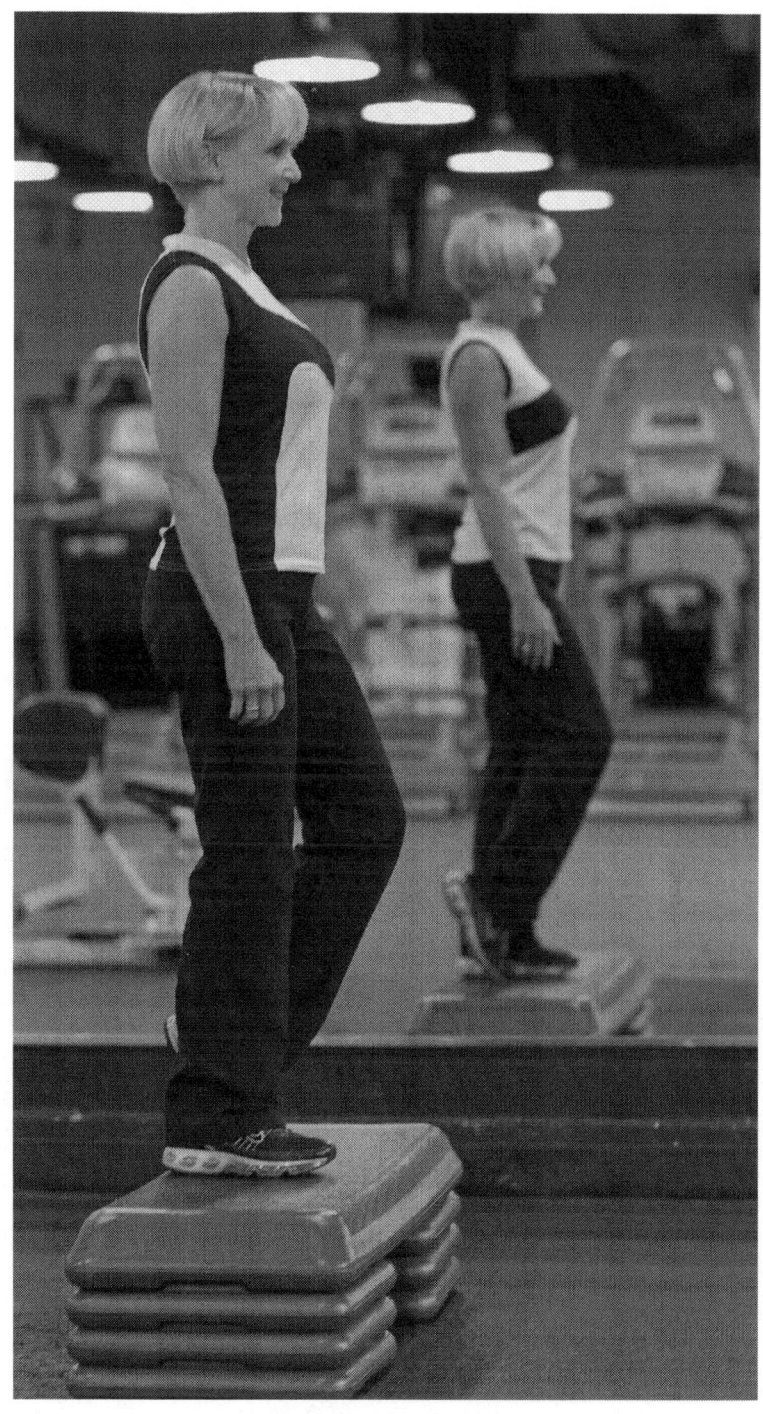

Bench Step-up – Middle

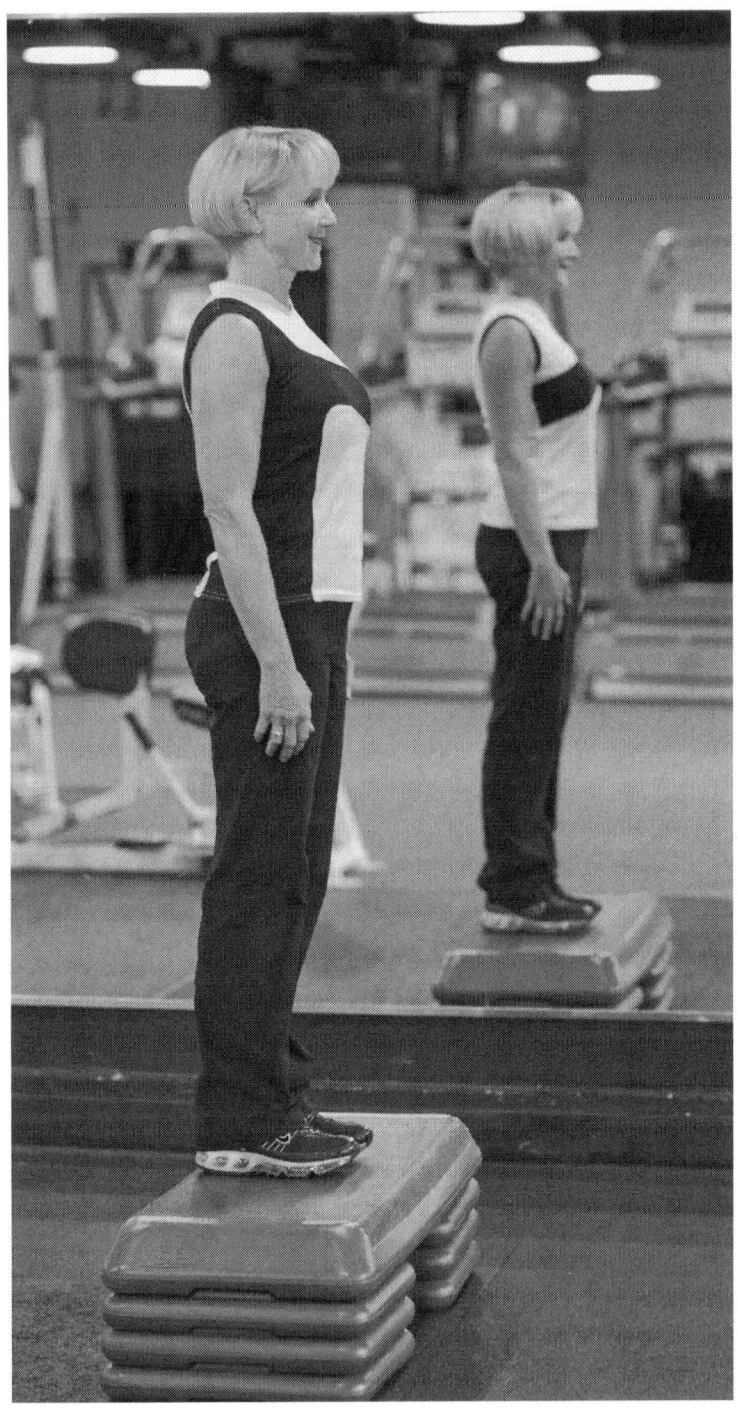
Bench Step-up – Finish

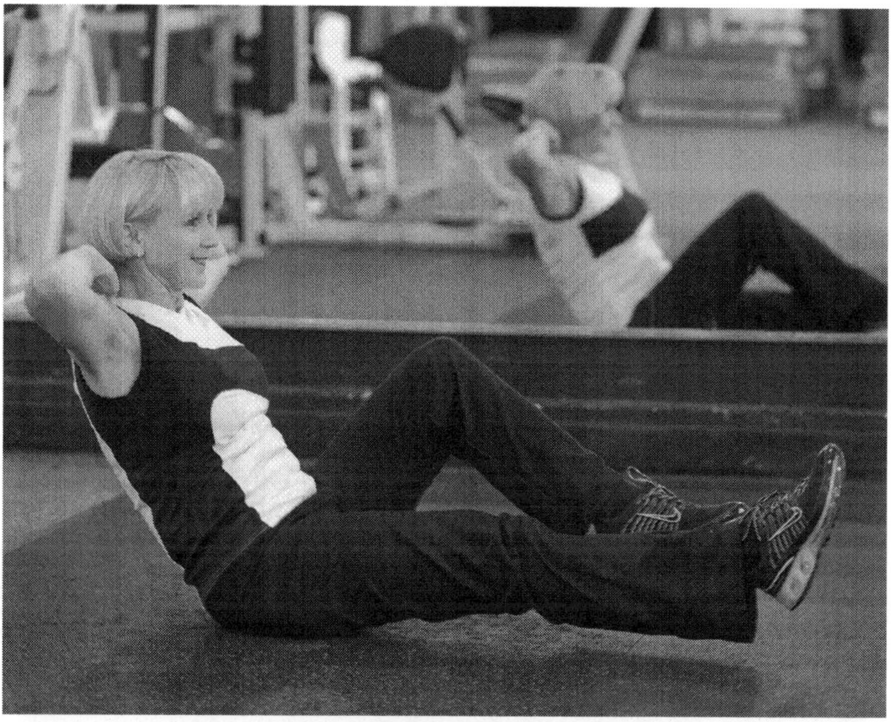

CURLING IRON: Strength Training

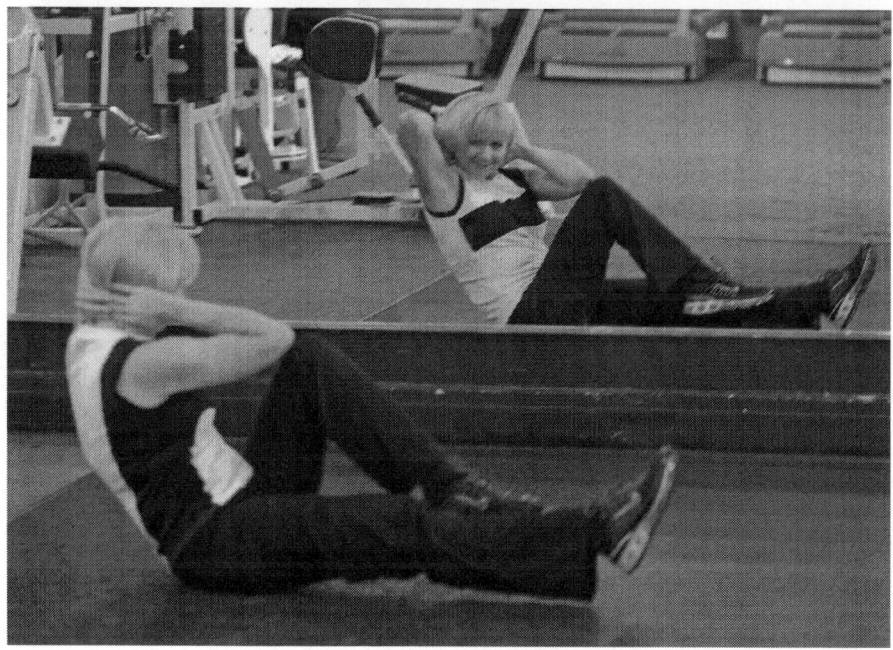

Bicycle – Start

Bicycle – Finish

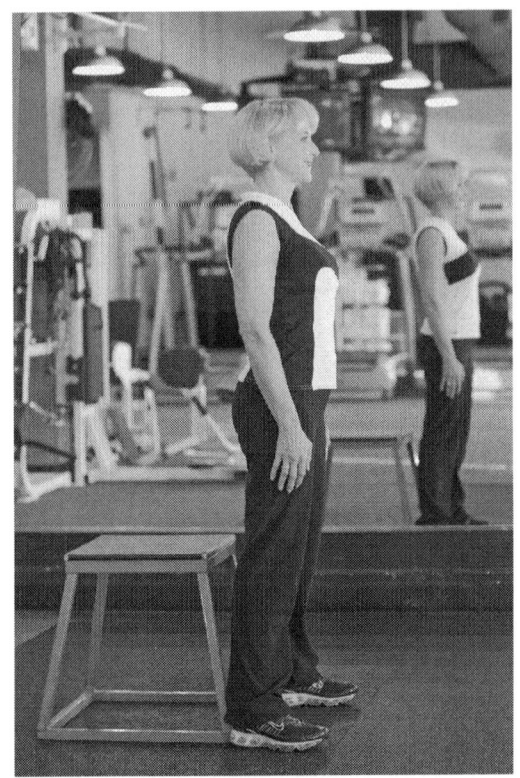

Box Squat – Start

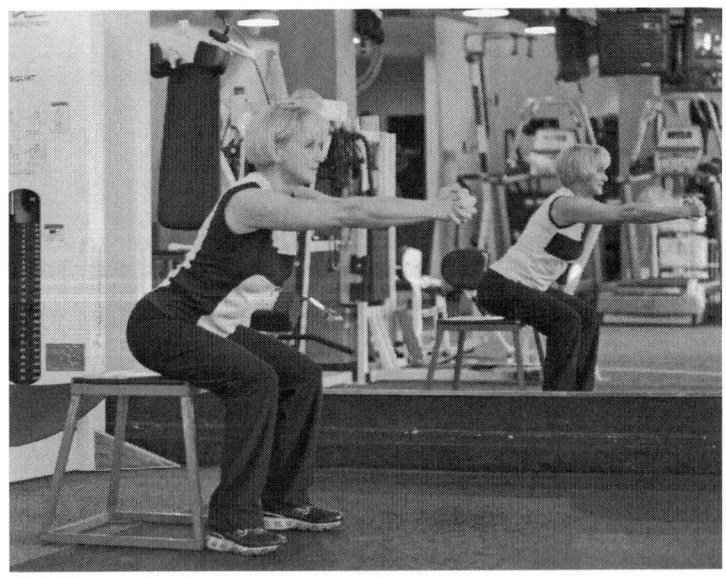

Box Squat – Finish

CURLING IRON: Strength Training

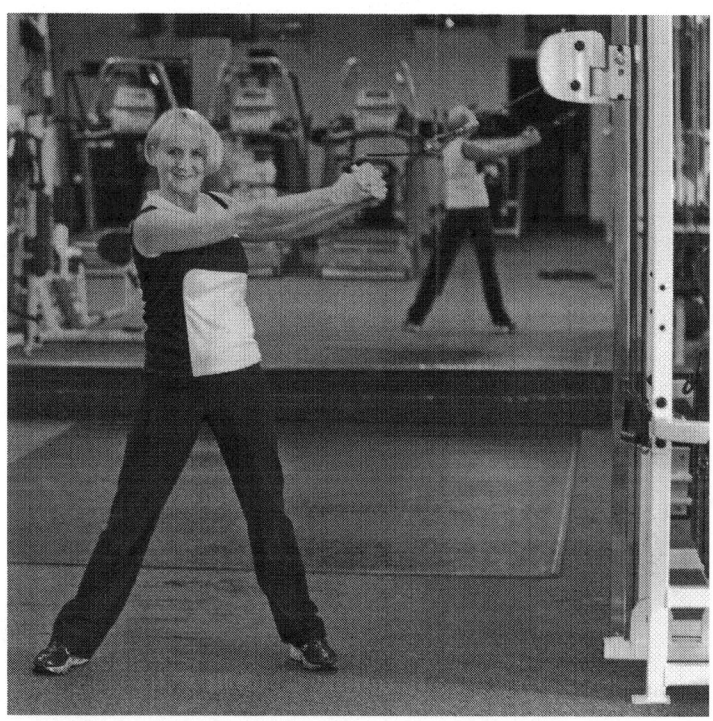

Lateral Wood Chop – Start

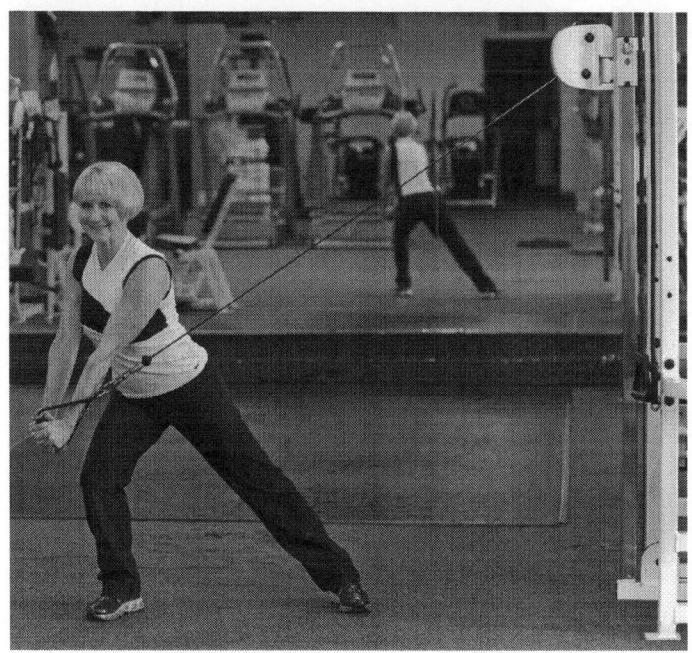

Lateral Wood Chop – Finish

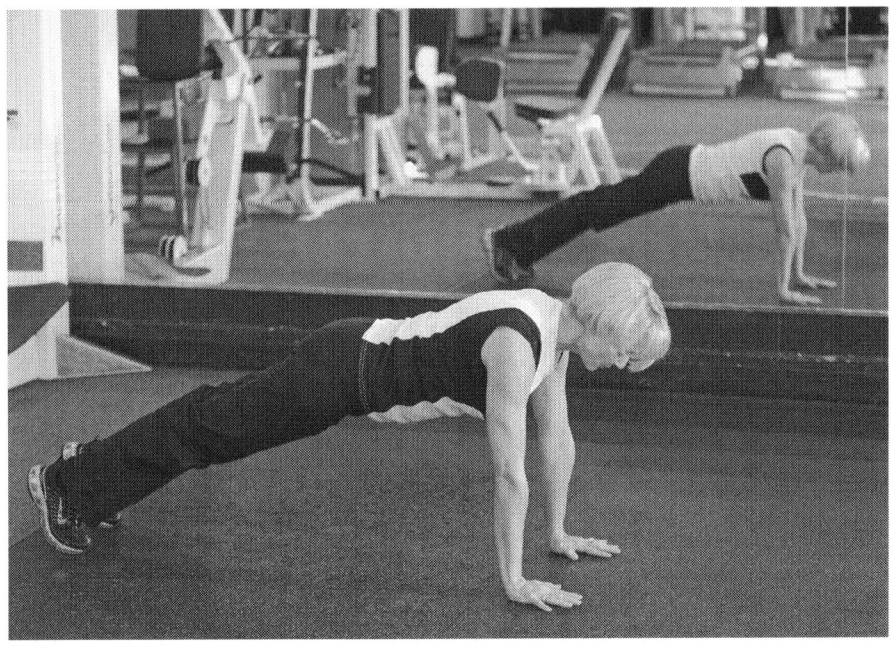

Push-up – Start

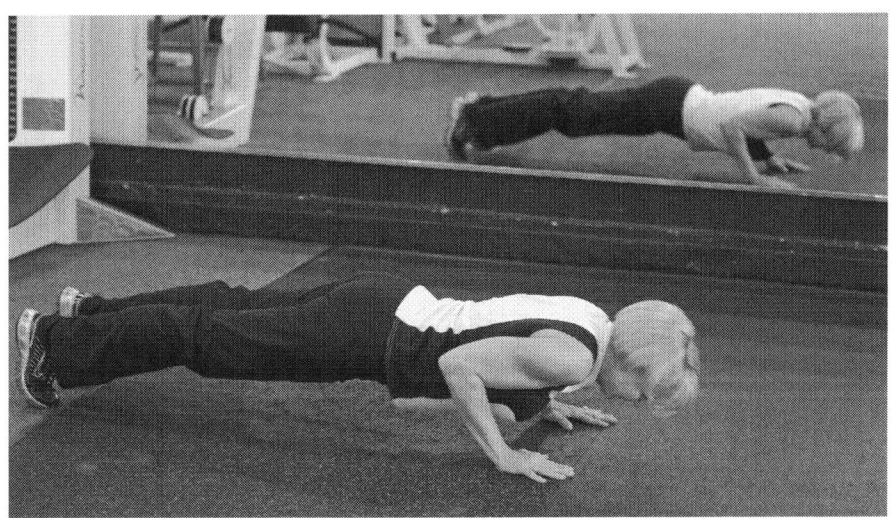

Push-up – Finish

CURLING IRON: Strength Training

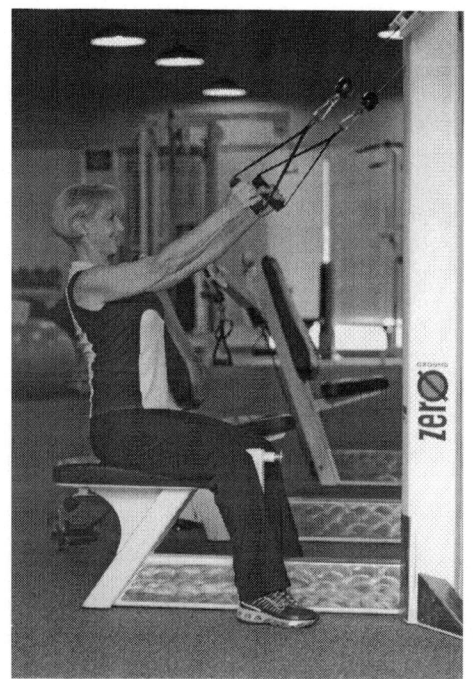

Seated Back Row – Start

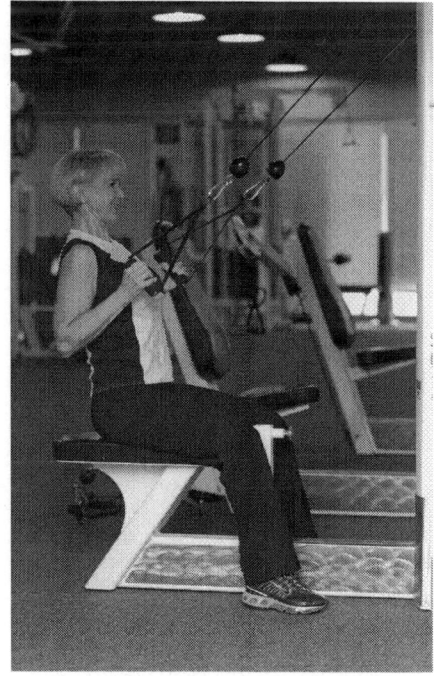

Seated Back Row – Finish

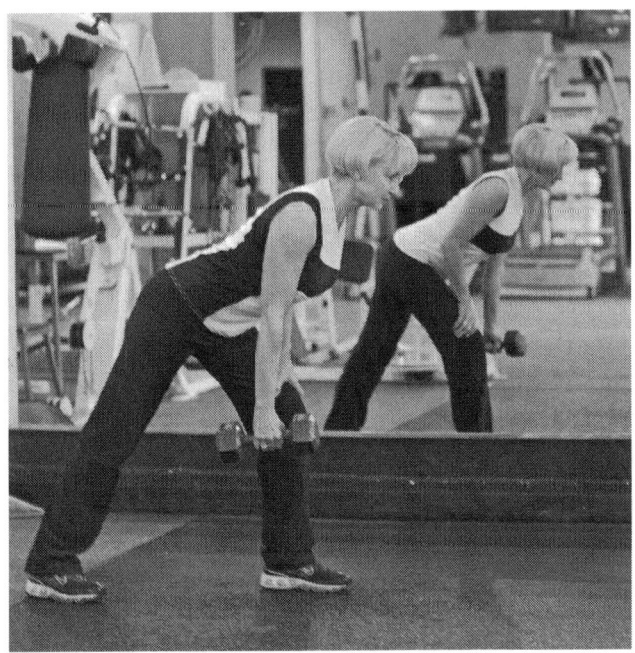

Standing Back Row – Start

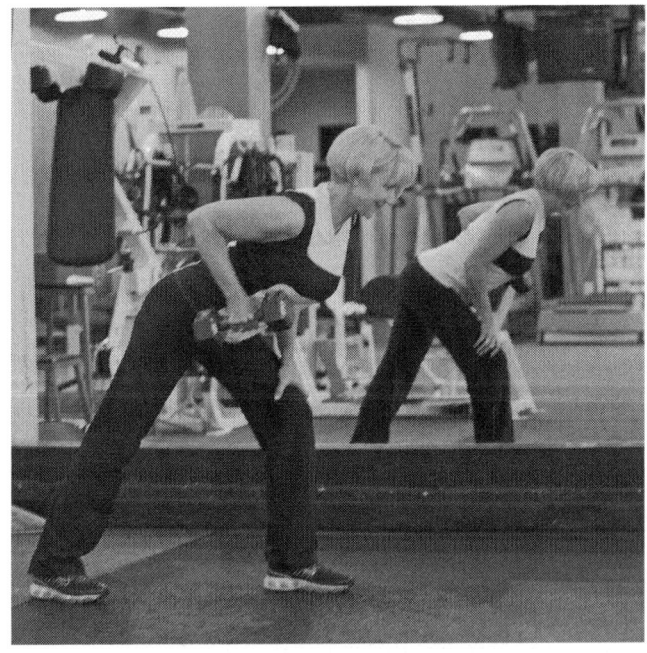

Standing Back Row – Finish

CURLING IRON: Strength Training

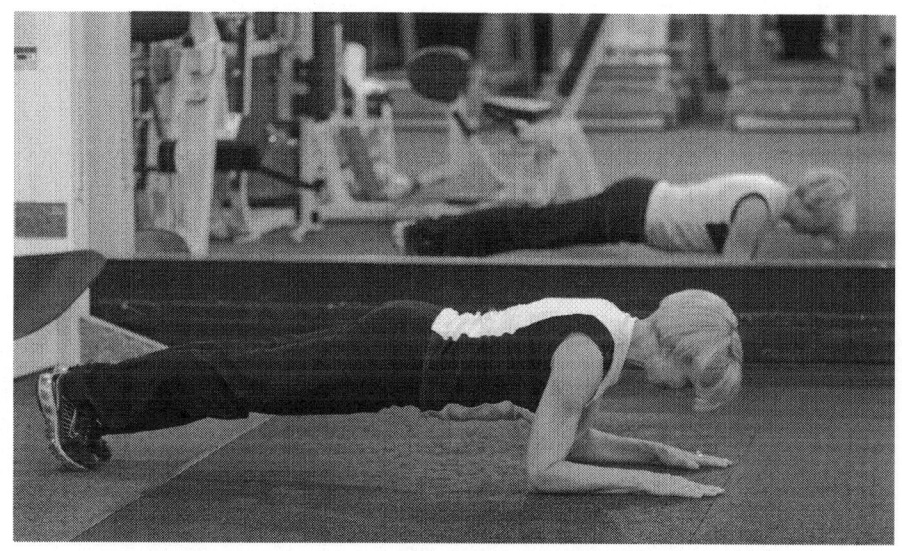

Static Plank

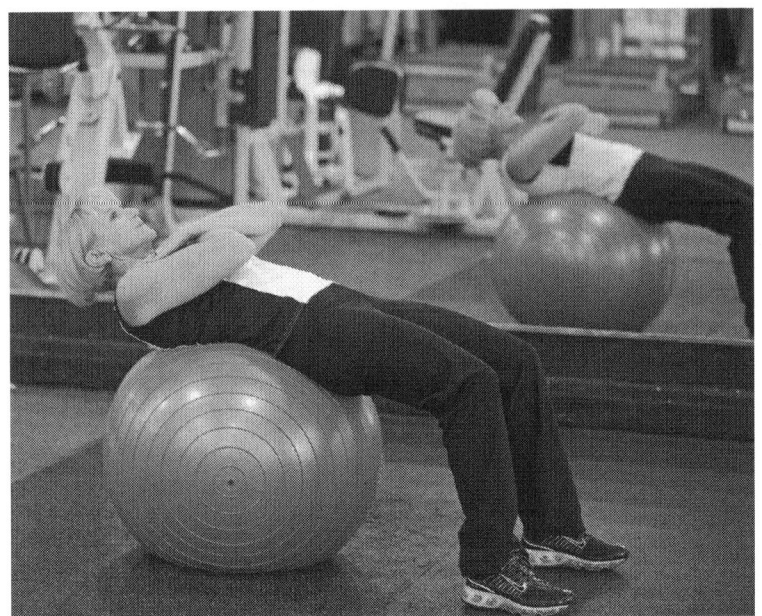

Swiss Ball Crunch – Start

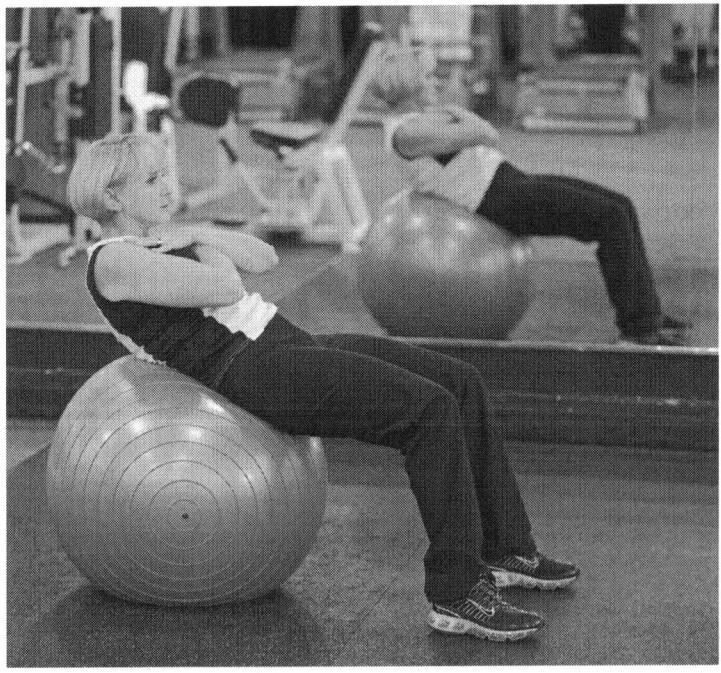

Swiss Ball Crunch – Finish

CURLING IRON: Strength Training

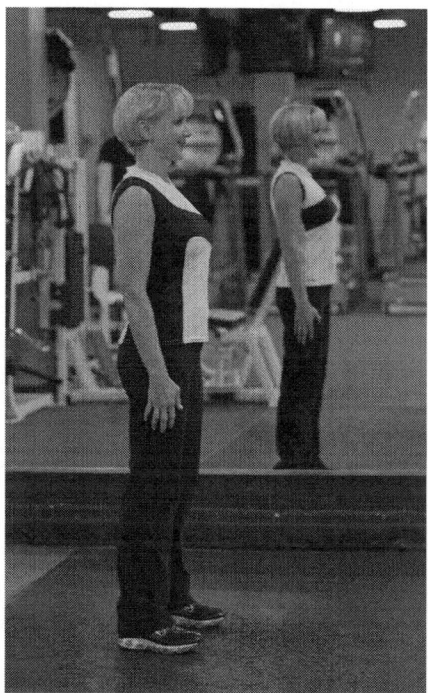

Walking Lunge – Start

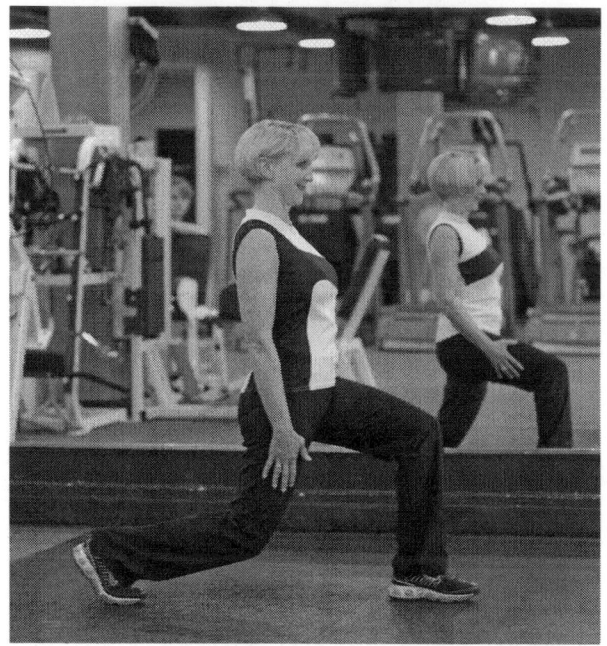

Walking Lunge – Finish

CHAPTER 6

THESE HEELS AND HILLS ARE KILLING ME:
What Women Do that Makes Their Bodies Hurt

Thoughts from Mary Jo:

I am five feet one inches tall. While there are many things I like about being short, I don't like standing in front of the judge's bench and he or she being barely able to see me, and vice versa. As a young lawyer, it bothered me enough that I wore three- and four-inch heels. I quickly learned to regret that. While carrying a very heavy trial briefcase up the stairs, I fractured a little bone in the ball of my foot. While the bone may have been small, it led to big problems. It was not a bone that could be set and I could not even walk. That led to the next mistake of allowing a podiatrist to remove it. That led to even further problems, which I still have to deal with today—some twenty-eight years later—all because I just had to wear those heels.

Now, while I no longer wear three- or four-inch heels, I do wear two-inch ones, which also sets me up for a plethora of problems. For one, it keeps my hips and calves tight. Hence, the title of this chapter. When you wear heels, the simple task of walking up a hill becomes difficult. When you are in flat shoes or athletic shoes after wearing heels, your calves burn and your hip flexors cry out for mercy.

I have a friend who has worn high heels for so long that she cannot even wear a flat shoe because it hurts so much.

You must be thinking that if it's such a problem, why do you wear heels at all? That is the question any sensible person would ask, but if you are like me, once again vanity gets in the way.

Women have several habits that can cause muscle aches and pains. The best action to take is to change those habits. However, if for whatever reason you can't or won't, there are some stretches you can do to minimize the pain.

Lu will explain what we are doing to our bodies when we...

1. Wear high heels
2. Wear a purse slung over our shoulder
3. Sit at a computer all day
4. Talk on the phone with the phone cradled on our shoulder
5. Cross our legs

Lu will try to get us to change these habits or, if not, at least learn to stretch.

What the Exercise Physiologist Has to Say: Lu Jurcova Phillips, M.S.

We are beautifully designed, with three shock-absorbing and energy-delivering curves in our spines, hips that tilt both front to back and side to side to accommodate the work of the legs, and shoulders that know almost no limit to their capacity to facilitate arm movement. When standing with our bare feet on the ground, we are the perfect combination of beauty and functionality.

Enter culture, and fashion, and our mothers, and bosses with deadlines (and let's not leave out our very own highly developed egos). Suddenly, the pretty curves in the last paragraph are exaggerated, function is reduced, and pain is an intimate friend. Let's look at a few of the things we do to ourselves, or allow others to do to us, that affect spinal curves, hip tilts, and shoulder carriage, and therefore our posture and our health.

High Heels

You and I both know that there are few things quite so aesthetically pleasing and transformative as lifting the heels just a few inches off the ground. Calves shift upward and tone and then taper to a smaller-appearing ankle, thighs firm, hips tilt slightly, the low back hollows out, the chest moves forward, and the shoulders fall back. It is powerful magic. But wielding such power comes at a price.

Including the three mentioned for the spine, there are a total of nine curves along the back of our bodies and the soles of our feet. These curves alternate to counterbalance one another, creating an undulating wave that distributes the effects of gravity and the forces created by our muscles. From the ground up, they are the ball, arch, and heel of the foot, the back of the knee, the sacrum (a triangular bone at the base of the spine), low back, midback, neck, and finally, the back of the head. Of these, the neck, the low back, the back of the knee, and the arch of the foot are maintained by muscles and other soft tissues. The other five are primarily maintained by the shape of the surrounding bones.

With this model of our anatomy in mind, let's revisit what happens when we slip into those high heels and change the angle and relationship of each of these curves with the ground.

The ball of the foot rolls forward and receives more weight. The muscles of the arch contract constantly to hold the position. The heel is held at its new elevation by the steady contraction of the calf muscles, which, because they also cross the knee joint, flex the knee forward. To pull the knee back into balance, the muscles on the front of the thigh will contract. One of these thigh muscles is attached to the front of the hip bone, and the contraction pulls it down. The back of the hip is pulled out and up, and this action forces the low back to curve more. The chest and rib cage are forced forward. The shoulders pull back to balance the chest, and the head and neck shift to stay on top of it all.

It's no wonder we're exhausted at the end of the day! To quote Ginger Rogers, she did everything Fred Astaire did, but she did it backward and in high heels.

I'm not suggesting a closet-clearing purge of everything but flats. I am saying that wearing high heels is now an informed choice, and we need to employ tools to counter the negative effects on our bodies each time we make that choice. Some tips:

Rotate. If it's not a requirement of your employment to wear a three-inch heel every day, choose outfits that allow you to change your heel height. Ideally, you should spend twice as much time walking barefoot or in flats as you do in heels.

Stretch regularly. If you put stretching on your to-do list and try to cram it in to your already over-full schedule, it will likely be the first item sacrificed. Give yourself the gift of a few minutes each day for the stretches in this chapter and you will be amazed at how much better you feel!

The High Heel Stretch – Either barefoot or wearing athletic shoes, stand facing a wall at arm's length and place your palms on the wall in front of you at shoulder height. Place your right foot six inches from the wall. Tuck your hips under so your pubic bone lifts toward your ribs. Flex the right knee and, keeping your torso vertical, press your hips and torso forward toward the wall, keeping your left knee straight and your left heel on the ground. Hold for thirty seconds. This should feel similar to the old calf-stretch we all learned in school or with a trainer. In this modification, you should feel a gentle stretch at the front of the left hip, in the left calf, and in the arch of the left foot. Release and repeat on the same side, and then do two repetitions with the left foot forward. Done correctly, this stretch will lengthen many of the muscles that are chronically contracted from wearing high heels.

You may find that you are unable to keep your heel on the ground when you begin this stretch. If you cannot, let it rise up to the point that you are feeling a gentle, effective stretch in the calf and the arch. Over time and with regular stretching, this will improve until you are able to perform the routine as described.

Lengthen and strengthen the core – Part of the posture of the high heel wearer (described above as the front of the hip being pulled down and the back of the hip being pulled out and up) is technically known as an anterior tilt of the pelvis. This forcing of the pelvis, comprised of the two hip bones and the sacrum, into an unnatural angle causes two important sets of core muscles to contract and shorten in order to protect the low back. One set of muscles, the lumbar paraspinals, is on the back and can be stretched by lying face down over an exercise ball. To properly and safely engage the stretch position, get on wide-spaced knees in front of the exercise ball and roll up onto

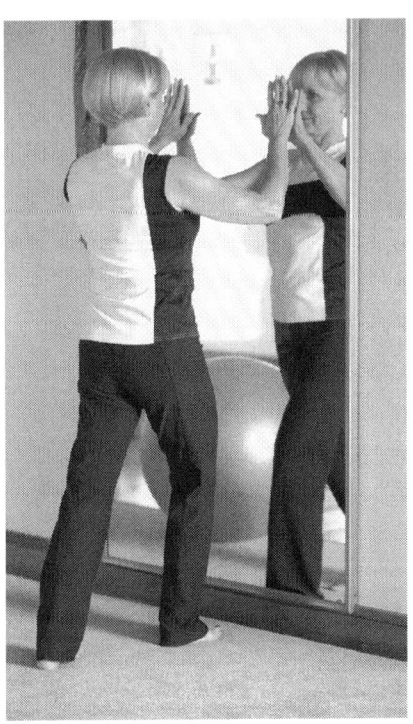

it slowly until your navel is balanced over the top of the ball. Keep either your widely spaced feet or hands on the floor to ensure stability. This is called the Lumbar Paraspinal or Low Back Stretch.

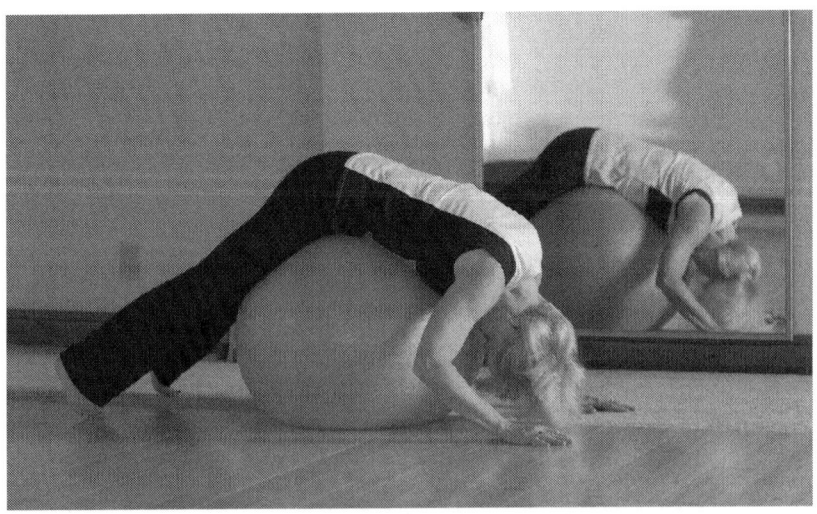

The second set of core muscles shortened by wearing heels, the iliopsoas group, is deep in the abdomen and acts to flex the hips. The High Heel Stretch, described above, takes the hip into extension and lengthens this muscle group nicely.

As discussed in the last chapter, strengthening these and the other muscles comprising the core is critically important to your overall well-being.

Crossed Legs

If I pause and listen for my mother's voice, I can still hear her say, "A young lady must *always* (emphasis hers) sit with her knees together or her legs crossed." I imagine each of you was similarly admonished. This advice helped us slip seamlessly into the cultural norm and is so deeply ingrained in our social behavior that it scarcely registers as a voluntary act. On a separate track, usually not taught by our mothers, we came to appreciate the beguiling effect of a timely uncrossing and re-crossing of the legs.

These two actions, holding the knees together and crossing the legs when seated, act on the hips and pelvic tilt in ways that can contribute to low back pain.

Here's why: holding our knees together is accomplished by large and small muscles on our inner thighs, collectively known as hip adductors. Each of these muscles attach to the thigh bone and along the lower edge of the pubic bone on the same side. The position of these attachments is important for our understanding of how these muscles can contribute to low back pain.

Recall that I said the pelvis, comprised of the two hip bones and the sacrum, is designed to tilt front to back and side to side. Please imagine a side view of a woman's skeleton and look at the hip joint, the thigh bone connecting to the hip bone. You will appreciate that this joint is the pivot point for the front-to-back tilt of the pelvis. There are sections of the hip bone that are in front of the pivot point, and sections that are behind it. Here is a diagram to make this a little more understandable.

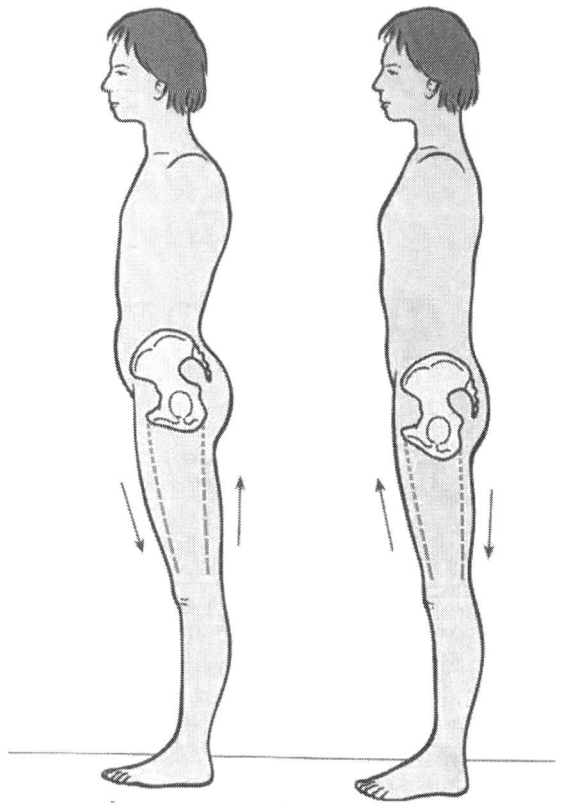

Muscles coming up from the thigh bone that attach to the hip bone in front of the pivot point will cause the pelvis to tip down in the front when they contract. Conversely, muscles coming up from the thigh bone that attach to the hip bone behind the pivot point will cause the pelvis to tilt down in the back when contracted. There are also muscles that attach to the pelvis from above that contribute to the ability to tilt the pelvis in this plane. The optimal functioning of this tilt, facilitated by long, supple muscles, contributes to our ability to walk and work and dance and enjoy sex. When any of these muscles are short and tight, all of those things are diminished.

The adductors, those muscles that bring our thighs and knees together when contracted, are at work and usually being overworked during most of our waking hours. The ladylike behavior of holding our knees together happens so frequently during each day that the adductors become shortened from the repetitive contractions. These shortened muscles, spanning from the thigh bone to their attachment on the pubic bone, cause the pelvis to tilt down in front when we are standing.

The sacrum, as part of the pelvis, tilts forward when the adductors pull down on the pubic bone, and this action is what can contribute to low back pain. The spine, with its three curves, sits atop the sacrum. When the sacrum tilts forward, the lowest of the three curves is forced to curve more in order to keep the torso upright. This exaggerated lumbar curve triggers the protective response of the core muscles I mentioned above.

Here are three different stretches for the adductor muscles. Choose one and work with it for two weeks, then move to one of the others. The rotation will focus on lengthening different fibers in the adductor muscles, as well as keep your routine fresh.

Standing Adductor Stretch – Stand with your feet double shoulder width apart. For some of you who are particularly tight, simply standing in this position will provide a sufficient stretch. If so, this is the perfect place to begin. Tuck your hips under, bringing your pubic bone up toward your ribs and hold the position for thirty seconds. Release the stretch and then repeat. Others of you may need to move further to engage a meaningful stretch. With hips tucked, allow your right knee to bend as you shift your weight to the right, until you feel the stretch in your left inner thigh. Hold for thirty seconds. Step out and then repeat, followed by the same routine on the opposite side.

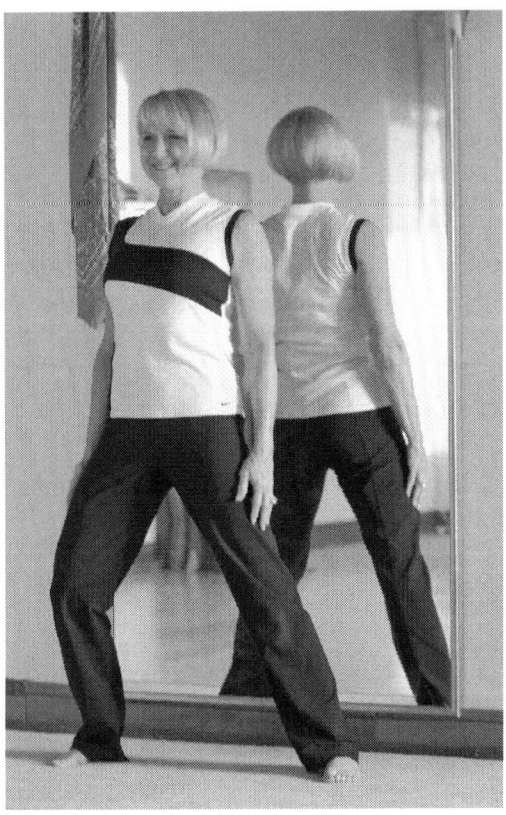

Seated Adductor Stretch 1 – Sit on the floor or a mat with your legs as far apart as comfortable and with your knees straight. Again, this position may be enough for some of you to experience a good stretch. For those who are ready for more, keep the back straight and lean forward from the hips. In each case, hold for thirty seconds, then release and repeat.

Seated Adductor Stretch 2 – Sit on the floor or a mat with your back straight and place the soles of your feet together, allowing your knees to fall outward toward the floor. Grasp your ankles and pull your feet gently toward you to engage the stretch and hold for thirty seconds. Release and repeat. For those wanting more, place your elbows on your inner thighs and press down as you lean forward from your hips, keeping your back straight.

THESE HEELS AND HILLS ARE KILLING ME

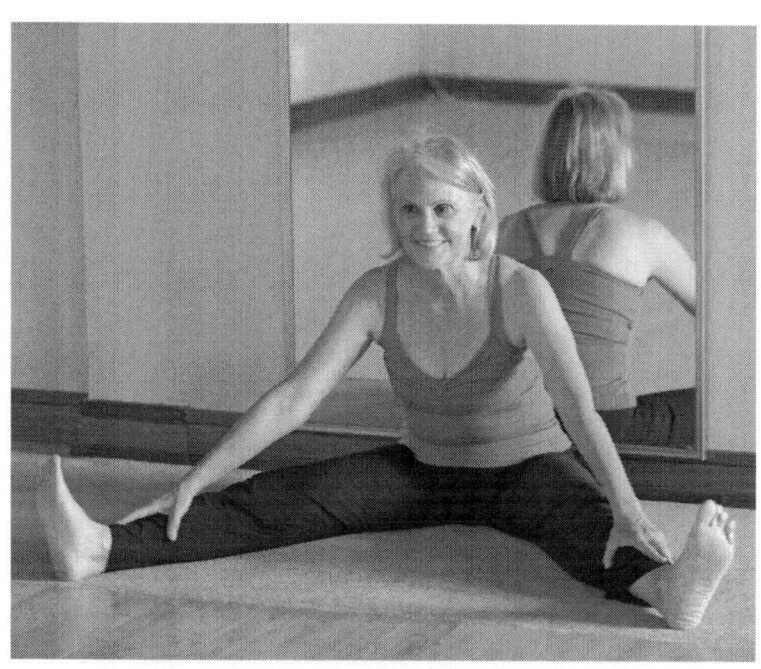

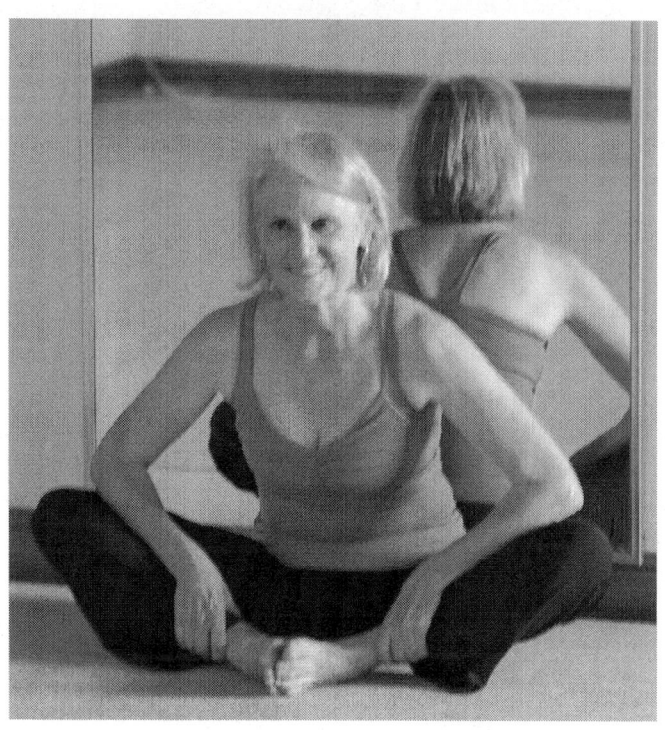

You will have noticed by now that my instructions for each of the stretches given in this chapter call for holding each repetition for thirty seconds. Many guidelines recommend ten to fifteen seconds, and you will certainly see improvement working at this duration. Current research shows that while holding a stretch for ten to fifteen seconds engages and lengthens the muscles fibers, staying engaged an additional fifteen seconds recruits a specialized area of the nervous system and causes beneficial changes to occur more rapidly. It's a sort of neuromuscular magic, and it is well worth the investment.

In the next two chapters, Mary Jo, Dr. Sahni, and Dr. DeLipsey will provide you with the knowledge—the wisdom, really—to eat in ways that will naturally help you shed pounds and feel great. But while you're still here, I'm going to tell you about:

Lu's Super-Duper-Appear-To-Have-Lost-Five-Pounds-Without-Even-Changing-What-You-Eat "Diet"

I've been discussing, in pretty technical anatomical language, the consequences of anterior pelvic tilt. Here's the scoop in plain language: the pelvis acts as a bowl or cradle for all the organs of the abdomen, and when the bowl tilts forward, all that stuff falls forward against the abdominal wall, making your tummy look bigger. Add to that the fact that a forward tilt in front means a backward tilt in back (i.e., it makes your butt look bigger because it is sticking out further), and you look five pounds heavier than you really are.

So the "Diet" is simply this—do the High Heel Stretch, the Lumbar Paraspinal/Low Back Stretch, and one or more of the Adductor stretches daily, and watch "five pounds" magically disappear.

We've talked about holding the knees together and how to counter the long-term consequences of that action, and now it's time to discuss the addition of crossed legs. All of the adductor contractions occur here as well, along with some new and interesting additional complexities.

In order to lift one leg up and over the other, the hip flexors on that side contract, along with a muscle in the side that lifts or hikes the hip bone, the quadratus lumborum, and some muscles in the abdominal wall called the internal and external obliques, which twist the trunk.

While most of us cross our legs in both directions, each of us has a preferred side, leading to a postural imbalance over time. We can overcome the effects of this imbalance by employing two simple stretches.

Side Bends – Assume the starting position for the Standing Adductor Stretch, including the hip tuck, then bend your torso to the right. Brace your right hand on your right thigh for added stability. Hold for thirty seconds, then release and repeat. Repeat the sequence to the left side. For a deeper stretch, extend the arm up and over the head on the side you are stretching.

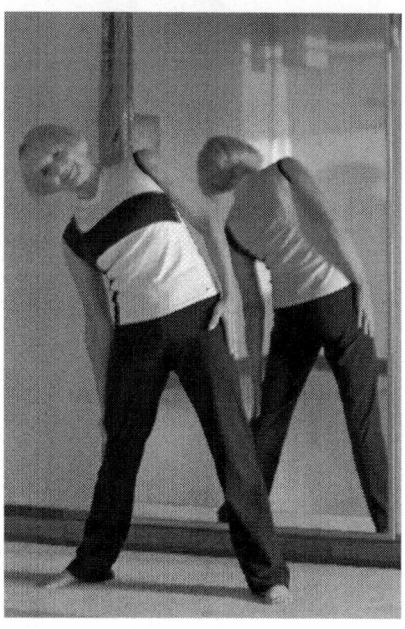

Side Twists – Stand with feet together and hips tucked. Rotate your trunk to the right while keeping your hips facing forward as much as possible. Hold for thirty seconds, then release and repeat. Repeat the sequence on the left side.

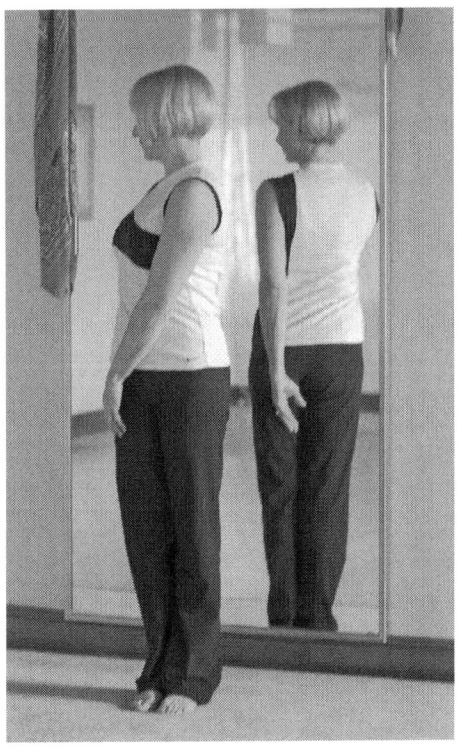

Seated versions of both these stretches may be performed safely in an arm or desk chair with a little experimentation. Remember to tuck your hips here as well.

Working at a Computer

Many of us, working in or out of the home, spend considerable time at a desktop or laptop computer. Taking a few minutes to think ergonomically and making small adjustments can help offset the impact on our posture of working with these now ubiquitous devices.

Your chair should allow you to sit fully against the back and not crowd or cut off circulation at the knees. If the seat portion is longer than your thighs, prop a pillow against the chair back, or use a different chair. The seat height should allow you to rest your bare feet flat on the floor. If not, adjust the height or acquire a footrest. Dangling in a chair that is too high causes circulation problems. Also, if you are working in an office and circumstances allow, by all means kick off those high heels. It's an opportunity to relax your calves. If your chair has arms and they are adjustable, move them so your arms hang comfortably down from your shoulders. We are each wonderfully (and differently) made, and upper arm lengths vary quite a bit. If your armrests are not adjustable and cause you to lift your shoulders, consider changing to an adjustable model or to an armless chair.

Standard desk and table heights have not changed to reflect the use of a keyboard, and most are simply too high. Ideally, you should be able to sit in a properly adjusted chair and have your arms hang straight down from your shoulders, with your elbows at a 90-degree angle when your hands are resting on the keyboard. If this is not the case, change the chair height to facilitate this proper shoulder and arm carriage, and add a footrest if necessary. Another option is to install a keyboard drawer, which will drop the keyboard to a more functional height.

With your furniture properly situated and sitting with good posture, your computer monitor should be at an elevation that has you looking at a point approximately one-third of the way down from the top of the screen. Any lower than that and you will be tilting your head down in order to see. This causes a strain on the small muscles at the back of your neck as they attempt to hold your head in this unbalanced position. A book or two of the right thickness placed under the monitor will solve the problem and, if they have interesting titles, can stimulate conversation.

Laptops are another matter entirely. For women on the go, they are a fantastic invention, but no matter where we place them, they are ergonomically problematic. There is simply no way to have proper monitor height and keyboard placement with a laptop. If this is your principal computer, consider getting a docking station with a regular monitor and keyboard for the fixed location where you use it most. If your primary use is on the fly, the stretches below will save you.

Long-term misuse of yourself with computers will cause you to slump, your shoulders to roll forward, your head to shift forward, and your neck muscles to shorten. Regardless of your circumstances, these few routines will help keep you from looking like Ebenezer Scrooge counting his money.

Mid-back/Chest Stretch – Stand in a doorway with your hands on the door frame at approximately shoulder height. Gently step forward until your arms are straight, reaching behind you to the door frame, and your body is vertical. You may have to rotate your torso to one side and then the other to accomplish this movement, depending on the width of the door frame. Hold for thirty seconds, then release and repeat. You will feel this stretch in the chest muscles, as an arching of the mid-back, and along the front of the arms. This routine will counteract both slumping through the torso and your shoulders rolling forward.

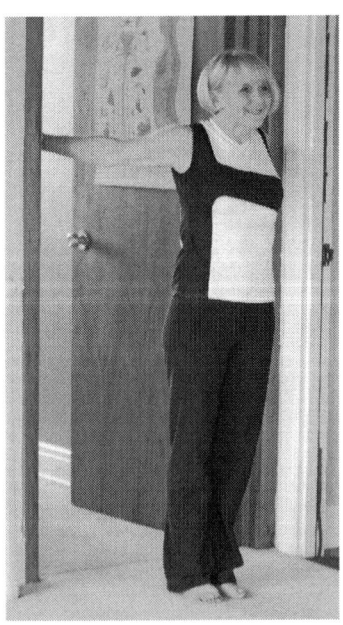

Forward Neck Stretch – Sit or stand with good posture, allow your head to fall forward, and bring your chin to your chest. Hold for thirty seconds, then release and repeat. You will feel this wonderful stretch at the back of your neck and down into your upper back. For a deeper stretch, lace your fingers together and place your hands at the back of the head. The weight of your arms will further lengthen the muscles. *Do not pull down on your head and neck with your arms.*

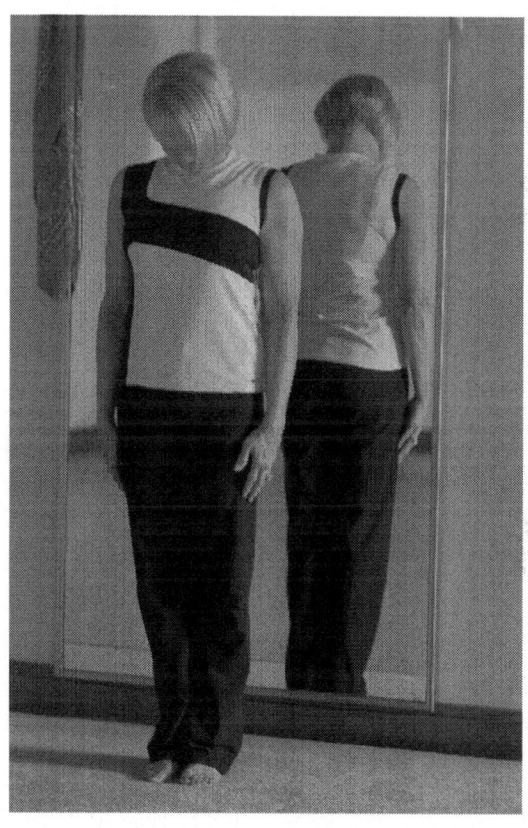

Many of us, when working at a desk or table for long periods, will unconsciously scoot forward to the front edge of our chair and lean into our task. This perching on our "sit-bones" at the lip of the chair will invariably cause us to move into an anterior tilt of the pelvis. This contributes to all the things we have discussed before about anterior pelvic tilt, and it can also cause us to get fuzzy-brained.

The "pump" for the fluid that bathes our brain and spinal cord is the natural rocking motion of our pelvis. When we lock ourselves into one position at the pelvis, the cerebrospinal fluid doesn't flow as well and can become stagnant, causing that fuzzy-headed feeling we've all experienced. When you notice a loss of mental clarity, pause and rock your pelvis front to back a few times, or get up from your chair and walk around for a minute or so. You'll notice a clearing of the mental fog almost immediately.

Telephones

The telephone, whether at home, the office, or on the go, is a major source of neck and shoulder problems. We are either elevating our shoulder and arm to hold the phone to our ear, or cocking our head to one side *and* elevating the shoulder to cradle the phone in order to free our hand for some multitasking event. And we spend more time on the phone now than ever before, resulting in sore necks, shoulder pain, and headaches.

Consider using a wireless headset for both your landlines and cell phones. It will free you from a vicious cycle of chronic contraction in the most vulnerable area of your spine. To restore lateral balance to the neck, do this easy stretch:

Side Neck Stretch – Sitting or standing with good posture, allow your right ear to drop toward your right shoulder. Keep the shoulder relaxed and low. Hold for thirty seconds, then release and repeat. You may deepen the stretch by placing your right hand over your left ear and allow the weight of the arm to lengthen the muscles. *Do not pull down with the arm.* Repeat the routine to the left side.

This is the appropriate juncture to mention a phenomenon I've noticed with my clientele. As cell phones have evolved into ever more complex communication devices, the computer posture we've just been discussing has now become associated with these new tools—with a vengeance. Instead of monitors and keyboards the width of our shoulders, we are now operating keyboards and

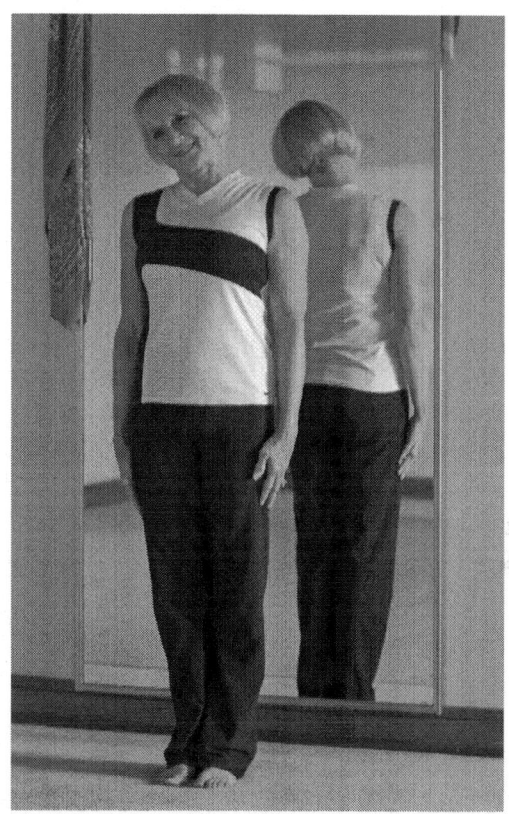

staring at monitors that are no more than three to four inches wide. The speed at which these postural syndromes are manifesting is truly alarming. If you use one of these marvels, you should be doing all of the computer and telephone stretches a minimum of twice per day. More is better.

Purses

Purses, fashion accessories par excellence, do double duty in the real world as utilitarian totes. In addition to what we carry for our own needs, the average purse contains a medical dispensary, a book's worth of lists, receipts for every purchase made in the last three months, entertainment, a snack and some mints, four pens, and way more computing power than the Apollo missions used to get to the moon and back. We're overloaded. If this doesn't describe your purse, you get a gold star. If it does, or if you're thinking, "That list isn't even close," it's time to regroup.

Inventory the contents of your purse monthly. File or throw away the paperwork. Return the remedies for your husband's cold last January to the medicine cabinet. Delegate. Get a small backpack for your child to carry his or her own entertainment. Recognize that you are not likely to read the paperback when you get a pedicure, since you haven't pulled it out the last three times. You get the idea.

It's important to do this periodic purge of unnecessary weight because it's burning up energy that could be better spent, and it's prompting a postural compensation. When a new client arrives for her initial evaluation, I can almost invariably identify her "purse shoulder" from the higher elevation relative to the other shoulder. And there is a direct correlation between the weight of the purse and the amount of compensatory elevation. Side Neck Stretches help here, too.

Finally, the hills. The literal and metaphorical hills in our lives alluded to in the title of this chapter will be much more readily scaled when you implement the changes I've outlined in our discussion. Do this simple test:

> Stand in bare feet on a level surface, next to something you can hold on to as needed for balance. Shift into an exaggerated anterior pelvic tilt—pubic bone down toward the floor and butt back and up. Lift your straight right leg out in front of you as high as you are able. Note the height, then release and return to the floor. Now reverse the tilt by tucking your hips under—lifting your pubic bone toward the ribs. Lift the straight right leg as before. How much higher were you able to lift your leg?

The change exemplified by this test, from unconscious dysfunction to conscious balance, is the heart of the matter. Physically, the shift translates directly into a longer stride length, with more power and more available energy reserves because we are using our resources efficiently and well. Mentally and emotionally, moving from balance imbues us with the confidence to be and do our very best.

PART THREE

FOOD FOR THOUGHT: NUTRITION

CHAPTER 7

YOUR MOTHER WAS RIGHT AFTER ALL:
Food for Life – Mindful Eating

Thoughts from Mary Jo:

As I grew older, the smarter my mother became. The first time I realized she was becoming smarter was my first year in college. She had had trouble keeping shoes on my feet my entire childhood. I always liked the way the grass felt under my feet on a spring day. I was walking across campus barefoot and stepped on a nail that went straight through my foot. This was an "Aha!" moment—"Oh, that's why she wants me to wear shoes!"

So, too, it is with what I eat. It was also while I was in college that she became smarter about what I should eat. The question that plagues me these many years later is: "How did she know?" She had no scientific study to guide her or book to tell her what was best. (She is now deceased, so I don't have the privilege of asking her or thanking her.) While my sister was always "little miss goody-two-shoes," the one thing that I had over her with my mother was that I would eat broccoli. I am eternally grateful to my mother that she had me eat it, for as an adult it is no chore.

When I came home from school, there were always plenty of fruits for me to choose to eat. That is not to say that I didn't eat my share of chips, but for those of us who ate lots of fruits and vegetables as youngsters, it is easier as adults to eat healthy.

So, what exactly does eating healthy mean? We are bombarded with "low-fat" diets or "low-carb" diets or "high-protein" diets, but the simple truth is that adhering to any "diet" is being on the wrong track. (We talk more about that in chapter 8.)

The truth is that eating to be healthy or as we should nutritionally requires a lifestyle change for most of us.

Alcohol

One word about alcohol: Alcohol requires much caution, because while some studies indicate that drinking in moderation can lower the risk of heart disease, more than that causes many more problems than it can possibly help. The research indicates that, for women, *one drink a day is the limit.*

Avoid Saturated Fats and Trans Fats

Because I am an attorney, I probably worry more about the possibility of being sued than most people, but at the risk of the fast-food industry suing, my mantra is **DON'T EAT IT!** The movie *Super Size Me* says it all. For those of you who have not seen it, I recommend that you do. It will change your view of fast food forever.

It's a documentary of a man who eats nothing but McDonald's food for thirty days and nearly destroys his health. In those thirty days his cholesterol went up sixty-five points, he gained 24.5 pounds, and his body fat went up 7 percent—all in just thirty days! At the end of thirty days, he not only had doubled his risk of heart disease, but he became depressed, exhausted, moody, had massive headaches, massive cravings, hardening of the liver, and no sexual desire.

We wonder why it's hard to get out of bed in the morning, or why we have no interest in a sexual relationship with our significant other, or why we always have headaches. The reporter in *Super Size Me* did for thirty days what many of us do over a lifetime.

Not only are saturated and trans fats packed with calories, they have no nutritional value. If you take a perfectly good piece of broccoli and deep-fry it, you have taken away all its value.

If there is a devil, there is no doubt that *he* invented saturated and trans fats. They taste so good and yet are so bad for you! These fats from Satan, as I call them, are linked to heart disease, stroke, diabetes, arthritis, cancer, and, of course, obesity.

But why? Why do these devilish foods wreak so much havoc, and why should they be avoided? Dr. Sahni will tell us.

What the Doctor Has to Say: Jyotsna Sahni, M.D.

We've got to eat to live, but conflicting information from books, magazines, TV, and even your own mother makes it hard to make good decisions about food. Whom do you trust? Fortunately, good advice about food is simple. It's about getting back to the basics.

There is absolutely no doubt that good health requires good nutrition. The food we eat provides the fuel and nutrients for our bodies to function optimally. So what's the best eating plan? I believe in food choices that are moderate, healthy, and balanced.

Food is more than nutrients that nourish your body; it can nourish your soul, too. Food is part of celebrations, holidays, religious rituals, and family traditions. Your individual taste and the tastes handed down by your family and cultural background make you unique. Honor your individuality, but temper your choices with the knowledge of how your diet will affect your health.

The good news is that you can train your palate over time for healthier cuisine while still respecting your own preferences. Tastes change over time anyway. After all, you know you are a grown-up when you would rather have crème brûlée for dessert than a Ding Dong.

Part of being a responsible adult is making responsible decisions about the care of your body. Some lucky people like healthy food from the get-go; others go kicking and screaming. Fortunately, most of us can be gently led to an improved way of eating. If you are starting with reasonably good health, there's no reason not to take baby steps. If you are suffering from illness, you may need to take a more extreme tack.

Tips For Improving Diet

Here are some tips for improving your diet.

Eat Mostly Fruits and Vegetables

Eat a (mostly) plant-based diet. There is a reason you have heard this a thousand times. Fruits and vegetables are full of water, fiber, vitamins, and minerals. They are good for your body and good for the earth, because growing them has much less detrimental impact on the environment than producing meat, poultry, and dairy. While the planet could handle this abuse in the past, it no longer can.

Fruits and vegetables are filling and generally low in calories. It's hard to over-eat spinach. Unlike most other foods, portion size doesn't matter much with vegetables. There's a health campaign going on for children that serves adults well, too. It's a daily goal that is fun and easy to understand: eat a rainbow every day. The idea here is simple: eat seven different-colored fruits and vegetables each day to get a wide variety of healthy phytonutrients. These plant-based nutrients can fight cancer, heart disease, and prevent the ravages of stress on the body. A general rule of thumb is that the more intense color a food has, the more nutritious it is. Think of deep red cherries and purple cabbage. "White" is not among the lovely rich hues in a rainbow, but is often found as a prefix to flour, bread, pasta, sugar, and potatoes. These "white" foods are best used sparingly. They have a high glycemic index and turn to sugar quickly in your body. High-sugar foods lead to a high blood sugar and may then lead to insulin resistance and type 2 diabetes, which are huge risk factors for heart disease. Of course, to any rule there are exceptions: enjoy cauliflower, onions, and garlic!

Drink Lots of Water

Drink lots of water. The earth is 70 percent water and so are our bodies. Most people roam around in a chronically dehydrated state. The first sign of dehydration is fatigue, and then comes the thirst, dry mouth, headache, and muscle cramps. We often confuse thirst with hunger and reach for a high-sugar treat to give us a boost of energy when what our body really wanted was simply a glass of water to fight feeling tired. Non-caloric (and decaffeinated) herbal teas and water with a wedge of lemon or a mint leaf will hydrate you healthily. Resist the temptation to drink your calories. Soda, energy drinks, sports drinks, coffee drinks, and sweetened teas can contain shocking amounts of sugar and calories. The brain simply does not register liquid calories. A Big Gulp at 7-Eleven is a whopping four hundred calories and twenty-nine teaspoons of sugar; a Venti Caffe Vanilla Frappuccino blended coffee with whipped cream at Starbucks contains a mind-boggling 430 calories! For the same number of calories, you could have four ounces of salmon, half a cup of brown rice, half a cup of steamed broccoli, and a dozen cherries for dessert. And you'd actually feel full (and be healthier)!

Avoid Processed Foods

Eat whole foods. Another way to say this is to avoid processed foods. We want our food to resemble its natural state as much as possible. When you choose the whole food version of the food you love, you will invariably get the high-fiber version. For example, it's better to eat the orange than drink the orange juice. Fiber fills you up, lowers cholesterol, lowers the effect of carbohydrates on blood sugar and insulin levels, and fights constipation.

Have you noticed how a bowl of oatmeal (steel cut oats are best) with a few walnuts and some berries sticks with you? It's a very different experience than a bowl of shredded wheat for breakfast. Shredded wheat doesn't even have added sugar, but it is so refined that it turns to sugar quickly in your body, and it's likely that you will feel hungry an hour later.

Fiber in Your Diet

Fiber is good. The average American gets twelve grams of fiber each day; the (minimum) recommendation is twenty-five grams daily! Processing foods not only depletes nutrients that fight disease, but also may add toxic chemicals like hexanes, which impair the nervous system. (Hexane is a toxic petrochemical widely used in processed foods.) Food that comes in boxes may be really old, as well as high in sodium and trans fat, among other unhealthy ingredients.

Read Food Labels

Read food labels. The ingredients on a food label are listed in order of decreasing amounts, which means that the first few ingredients are most plentiful. Chances are if you can't pronounce or spell the ingredient, it's not good for you; therefore, limit your consumption of packaged items. Even the packaging itself pollutes the earth; a banana peel is a biodegradable container provided to you by Mother Nature herself.

Eat Fresh, Seasonal Food

Eat fresh, seasonal, and local as much as you possibly can. Fresh food means your food is not frozen, dried, or in a jar or can. Food that's in season will be fresher, tastier, healthier, and less expensive. If the origin of the food isn't labeled, ask the store manager where it came from. Ideally, it is grown within a day's drive to your grocery store or at least on your own continent. There are some wonderful things about living in a global market, but fresh food should come from close to home. Food that has been cultivated for long-distance shipping is often picked green and then chemically ripened. Often pesticides that are prohibited in the United States are still being used in other countries.

Clearly, our health may be comprised by our food choices, but so too is the health of the earth. For example, our demand for winter fruit has led to deforestation in South America. Instead of long-distance imports, explore farmers' markets in your area. Get to know the people who cultivate local crops and put dinner on your table. Visit the farms, see how they treat the plants and animals there, and even harvest your own fruits and vegetables. There's nothing fresher (or more fun!) than picking your own apples in the fall or peaches in the summer. When there's a local bumper crop of something you love, buy in quantity and freeze it.

If you can grow it yourself, do it! Tomatoes, squash, and herbs are easy to grow in the ground or even in container gardens. By planting the seeds, nurturing the plants, and watching them grow, you become even more connected to the food you eat.

Lean Proteins

Eat lean proteins. Protein can come from beans, soy foods, quinoa, fish, eggs, dairy, and the leanest cuts of poultry and red meat. Again, choose vegetarian options most often. Numerous studies have linked meat consumption with heart disease, blood clots, and breast and colon cancer. Less is more when it comes to meat.

Eat Healthy Fats (Sparingly)

Eat healthy fats (sparingly). Fats are where the flavor is and they lend a creamy, satisfying mouth-feel to food. But they can be unhealthy if they are saturated. Saturated fats are solid at room temperature, so we're talking about butter, cheese, bacon, ice cream, milk fats, and meat fats. If you can cut it off your rib eye steak, it's a saturated fat. Saturated fats raise the LDL or "lousy, loser" cholesterol, which can lead to clogged arteries. That's different than olive oil (organic extra virgin is my choice), which will never hurt your cholesterol because it's a mono unsaturated fat. Healthy fats also include avocados, nuts, and organic coconut and expeller-pressed canola oil. Omega-3 fats are especially good for your health and may reduce heart disease, stroke, depression, Alzheimer's disease, cancer, and inflammation. They come from fatty fish like wild salmon, halibut, and sardines, as well as nuts and flax.

Also avoid trans fat. Trans fat is a fat that does not occur in nature (partially hydrogenated fat/oil). It is often used in baked goods and fast foods. Some examples of trans fat foods are potato chips, doughnuts, margarine or many salad dressings.

Portion Size of Fats

Be especially vigilant of portion size when it comes to fats. Sadly, they are very high in calories. Fats are more than twice the calories of proteins and carbohydrates, with nine calories per gram versus four calories per gram in proteins and carbohydrates. Half a cup of nuts and half a cup of olive oil, both healthy fats, contain five hundred calories!

Reduce Sugar Intake

Reduce your sugar intake. According to the USDA, the average American consumes an astonishing 156 pounds of sugar each year. Clearly, it makes good sense to cut back. Your palate will adjust to less sweetness with time. Often, though, people use sugar substitutes instead. Saccharine, aspartame, and Splenda are common, but I don't like them. I don't trust any food that has been invented in a laboratory. Studies have show that these artificial sweeteners increase obesity, heart disease, and other serious illnesses. You are actually better off eating real sugar than these substitutes! I would rather you use honey, maple syrup, molasses, brown sugar, agave nectar, fruit juice, and evaporated cane juice, which actually contains trace nutrients that are normally removed from fully refined sugar. Unfortunately, these healthy options all contain calories. For those of us who are battling the bulge, I prefer Stevia, an herbal product, as a non-caloric sweetener.

Eat Less Salt

Eat less salt. Most Americans get too much salt in their diets. Some comes from the salt shaker, but huge amounts are hidden in processed foods because salt is a good preservative and can keep a food on the shelf longer (another reason to avoid processed foods!). The trouble is that wherever salt goes, water follows. This is why, for many of us, the day after we have a bag of pretzels, our rings and shoes are tight and our weight is up several pounds. Fluid retention is more than uncomfortable; it can lead to high blood pressure, which can then lead to heart disease, stroke, and kidney disease.

Salt does enhance the flavor of food, but like many condiments, it is an acquired taste. We can acculturate our taste for less salt and within weeks notice a change in our desire for it. Mediterranean sea salt is unrefined, has a little less sodium, and is higher in a few other minerals than regular table salt; it is what I use in my own cooking. I encourage you to learn to cook with a wide variety of spices and herbs and less salt. Not only do these add loads of taste to your meals, but they may also have health benefits. For example, cinnamon may help you raise your HDL, or "healthy" cholesterol. Turmeric reduces inflammation in the body, and ginger aids with digestion. Nature has many more flavors than Baskin-Robbins. Have fun and experiment!

Portion Size in General

Be mindful of your portion size. Everyone, including professionals, underestimates the size of portions. You may be very surprised to learn how small a serving size truly is. Most of us overeat, and restaurants encourage this unhealthy behavior. When we understand appropriate portion size, it's easy to understand why one-third of America is obese and two-thirds is overweight. We eat too much and eat the wrong foods.

Ironically, we are simultaneously overfed and undernourished. For example, one serving of fruit is a medium-sized apple, half a banana, or just four ounces of fruit juice. One serving of vegetable is half a cup of cooked broccoli or one cup of loose leafy greens. One serving of protein is four to six ounces of tofu, chicken, fish, or steak. This can be visualized as roughly a deck of cards. Most restaurants serve six to nine ounces of chicken and seven to sixteen ounces of steak. One serving of grain is one slice of bread, half a cup of dry cereal, or half a cup of cooked rice or pasta. One serving of dairy (ideally, low-fat or nonfat) is one cup of milk or yogurt or one and one-half ounces of cheese.

The traditional food pyramid put forth by the USDA in the 1960s has made us sick and fat. Topple it over! Make fruits and vegetables the base, with nine servings a day, followed by only four grains, two servings of low-fat dairy, and three servings of lean protein, and eat oils, salad dressing, mayonnaise, nuts, and sweets stingily. Of course, your individual needs may vary a bit depending on your height, body frame, age, exercise habits, medical concerns, desire to lose weight or maintain weight, as well as your unique metabolism. Everyone is different, but the principles here apply to all.

You don't want to be starving when you sit down at the table. It takes twenty minutes for your stomach to give your brain the message that it's full. When you're over-hungry, you tend to eat too fast and miss the critical message of satiety. As a result, you are more likely to overeat. In addition, when you eat too fast, you may not chew properly. It may sound incredibly obvious, but not chewing your food well enough leads to poor digestion, burping and belching because of swallowed air, and a stomachache. Also, when you're famished, your blood sugar may drop, making you feel weak, dizzy, and irritable, and might give you a headache. These symptoms may occur before your stomach growls. Recognize them and feed yourself well.

Eat smaller meals with greater frequency. Have three modest meals and two small snacks each day, or four to five small meals. This simple formula helps prevent you from being starving or from overeating. Since calories are actually consumed with the work of digestion, eating more often boosts the metabolic rate of the body. It may also keep blood sugar levels more stable, thereby keeping energy levels and mood more even. Since meals are relatively small, having healthy snacks on hand for hunger attacks if they should occur can preempt an unhealthy binge at a vending machine or fast-food joint.

Stop eating when you are gently satisfied, not when you are full. It's interesting to me that a lot of my patients who say that they are never hungry for breakfast simply overeat their dinners. When they eat a smaller dinner, they feel less sluggish in the evening, sleep better, and over time find themselves developing an appetite for breakfast.

When you're eating, just eat. If you have been in the habit of overfilling your belly at mealtime, it takes some time and lots of attention to change old habits.

Avoid Multitasking During Your Meal

Avoid the modern habit of multitasking during mealtime. You should be sitting at a table while you're eating, not in the car driving, on the couch watching TV, or talking on the phone. When you can actually pay attention to the food and the effect it's having as you eat it, you will discover things you don't know about yourself and the foods you choose. Your taste may have changed over time; a food you thought you liked may not be satisfying to you now.

Very often people realize that when they pay attention to the eating process they need a far smaller quantity of food to satisfy their hunger. Some foods (like fruits and vegetables, which are rich in prana, or life force) may give you a feeling of being light and healthy, whereas other foods (like three-day-old pepperoni pizza) may leave you feeling heavy and down. When you pay attention, you will note the subtle differences in the energy of the foods you eat.

Food may taste different and feel different if you are eating while having an argument with your spouse or child at the dinner table. There may be differences depending where you are in your menstrual cycle. Without observing yourself, you won't know what you are really hungry for. Sometimes the hunger is for a good night's sleep, or laughter, or a hug, rather than a pint of Ben and Jerry's ice cream.

Buy Organic When Possible

Avoid pesticides, herbicides, antibiotics, hormones, additives, preservatives, pathogens, and genetic modifications. One way to make sure your food is clean and safe is to buy organic. The U.S. government has stringent guidelines for food producers to qualify for this certification. Studies have shown that organic food is also more nutritious. If you have a choice, organic is usually the better one. It has more good stuff, less bad stuff, and usually tastes better too.

Since organic food tends to more expensive, it may not be practical or possible to eat only organic. There are some foods that you shouldn't compromise on, however. According to the Environmental Working Group, this list is known as the "dirty dozen": peaches, apples, bell peppers, celery, nectarines, strawberries, cherries, kale, lettuce, imported grapes, carrots, and pears. Eating other fruits and vegetables that are not organic is less critical.

Food also should be literally clean. Always wash food well (before cutting it) to remove dirt, bacteria, and pesticide and herbicide residue. Peel the skin off wax-coated non-organic produce such as cucumbers, and throw away the outer leaves of lettuce and cabbage. Even organic fruits and vegetables need to be washed well.

Avoid Mercury

Avoid mercury. Mercury toxicity is a health hazard that is becoming increasingly recognized. One government analysis shows that each year 630,000 children are exposed to potentially unsafe mercury levels in the womb. Eating canned tuna is the biggest cause. In March 2004, the FDA and the EPA issued the first ever joint advisory on this topic. Burning coal is the largest cause of mercury in the oceans, lakes, and rivers, and the levels keep rising.

The most common dietary source of mercury is large fish. Here's how it works: the large predator fish eat the medium-sized fish, which eat the small fish, which eat tiny mercury-containing organisms. As a result, the mercury becomes more concentrated as you move up the food chain. The large predator fish—like tuna, swordfish, shark, king mackerel, marlin, and tile fish—are high on the food chain and also high in mercury. Mercury is a heavy metal that is a neurotoxin; it goes to the brain, nerves, and spinal cord. Subtle symptoms of mercury toxicity include fatigue and depression. Severe symptoms of mercury include tremors and dementia. Who hasn't had a fatigued and depressed day? Limit the large mercury-rich fish to only two or three times a month.

If you consume lots of these fish, consider checking your mercury level. A blood test provides an easy screening tool, but will only reflect the previous six weeks or so, not an overall mercury body burden. More sophisticated testing is harder to come by, but is available if necessary. The smaller wild fish like salmon, sardines, and anchovies are your best choice. On the other hand, farm-raised salmon, which includes "Atlantic salmon," has been found to contain significant quantities of four serious health contaminants.

Conclusion

Too often, a patient with a serious disease asks me, "Why did this happen to me?" The answer, in part, is poor diet. Did you know that cancer will soon overtake heart disease as the number-one cause of death in the United States? The consumption of enormous quantities of convenience food, along with the demand for greater and greater corporate profits, has led to the deterioration and poisoning of our food supply. While I don't advocate a radical approach to healthy eating, it's wise to keep this information in mind as you make your food choices.

Finally, have an attitude of gratitude. Be grateful for your food. Sadly, there are many parts of the world where food is scarce, even here in the United States, the "breadbasket" of the world. Taking a moment to feel grateful for the food on your plate helps you slow down, appreciate your life, and savor that food. Break bread with family and friends. After all, nourishment is more than good nutrition; it's also about the people you love and those who love you.

CHAPTER 8

CHOCOLATE IS A MAJOR FOOD GROUP, ISN'T IT?
Healthy Weight Strategies

I have this theory that chocolate slows down the aging process. It may not be true, but do I dare take the chance?
—*Anonymous*

Thoughts from Mary Jo:

My friends know that I would rather eat chocolate than any other food. For me, it is a major food group! For you, it may be French fries, movie popcorn, or hamburgers. My mother used to say "thirty seconds on the lips, thirty years on the hips."

If you want to lose weight, dieting is not the answer. There is a reason the first three letters in the word "diet" are D-I-E.

There are low-fat/high-carb diets, there are low-carb/high-fat diets, there are liquid diets, but the truth is that they do not work for most of us. Sure, we can lose a great deal of weight on any of those diets, but what happens when we start eating again the way we used to? We gain all the weight back, and sometimes more.

We have to make permanent lifestyle changes. But there's good news.

Did you know that scientists have found that your pleasure receptors are maxed out after just three bites? So one of your plans might be to share one of those forbidden foods with someone and go for those first three bites. Or you might, when the meal is served, cut it in half and ask for a to-go box up front. At home, you might serve on smaller plates.

The other component of healthy weight strategies is to be aware that you shouldn't just concentrate on the number of calories you take in, but also the exercise you are getting.

If you just lose weight without exercise, you are more than likely losing muscle along with fat. To maintain your weight, you should exercise a minimum of three times a week for a minimum of thirty to forty-five minutes. To lose weight, you should exercise five or six days a week for a minimum of thirty-five to forty-five minutes. This will keep your metabolism revved up all week. (By the way, you do not have to do all thirty-five to forty-five minutes at one time.) Studies have shown that even three ten-minute periods of movement can help in weight loss. The next time you have only ten or fifteen minutes in your day, don't use that as an excuse not to move. Take a walk around your block or your office building.

The last thing I want to mention is to become aware of your eating and, if you are going to eat or drink something that is not particularly good for you, make it a conscious decision and plan the rest of your meals accordingly. For example: one glass of wine is one hundred calories or more. If you drink one glass of wine a day, you might consider eliminating it. Just that change alone is equal to one pound of fat in a year. Small changes over a long period of time can make big differences.

Bon appétit!

What the Psychologist Has to Say: Jan DeLipsey, Ph.D.

The Simple Weight-Loss Plan

If your goal is to lose weight, this chapter will teach you how. Healthy weight loss is doable, although from the number of books, magazine articles, talk-show programs, and hordes of overweight Americans, you would think that shedding pounds was one of the great mysteries of the cosmic universe.

There is no question that most of us need to lose weight. There is no question that being overweight invites many undesirable consequences, ranging from increased risk for serious illnesses to just feeling bad and unattractive. There is no question that most of us want to lose weight. The real question is, how do you do it and how do you keep it off?

The mechanics of losing weight are simple: the calories you burn must be greater than the ones you consume. Here is a fact: anyone—absolutely anyone—who is overweight can lose weight.

Body Composition: Bones, Muscle, and Fat

A successful weight change plan starts with a good understanding of your body's composition, which is the proportion of fat to muscle and bone. Knowing the percentage of fat, muscle, and bone will allow you to establish your ideal weight range, guide you in developing a nutritional plan, and help you tailor an effective exercise plan.

Muscle burns calories; fat does not. A 150-pound woman with 40 percent body fat can consume the same amount of calories as a 150-pound woman with 28 percent body fat, but the latter will not gain weight because her more muscled body naturally burns more calories. Simply put, the lady with more muscle has a high basal metabolic rate (BMR). I'll go into more detail about BMR later in the chapter.

It is important to know your body's composition when you begin your weight-loss plan and to focus your exercise plan on increasing muscle mass while decreasing body fat.

Body Mass Index

Body mass index (BMI) is an easy and quick estimate of weight and height to lean body mass. BMI is a rough estimate, so it is best used as a screening tool. BMI is not to be confused with BMR (basal metabolic rate). The former refers to your body's composition; the latter refers to the amount of energy expended by your body when in a neutral state. You need to know them both.

The Centers for Disease Control publishes an automatic BMI calculator and tables of BMI ideal weight ranges on the Web.[6] If you want a rough estimate of your BMI right now, use the following formula:

Weight in pounds divided by height in inches, squared, then multiplied by 705

Example: A 150-pound woman who is 65 inches tall
65 squared is 4,225; 150 ÷ 4225 = 0.036; 0.036 x 705 = 25.0

BMI	Weight Status
Below 18.5	Underweight
18.5 – 24.9	Normal
25.0 – 29.9	Overweight
30.0 and Above	Obese

BMI STATUS TABLE

(Centers for Disease Control and Prevention)

Looking at the Centers for Disease Control table above, our sample lady would be teetering between the normal and overweight category. BMI is best used only as a screening tool because many other factors also "weigh" in this calculation. BMI should be considered an overestimate if one has a good amount of lean muscle and an underestimate if one has a good amount of fat.

For example, if our 150-pound lady were a muscle-bound athlete, she could conclude from this screening that she is in a normal weight range. However, if she were sedentary with noticeable abdominal fat, she should conclude that she is overweight and at risk for health problems.

Although it is helpful to know your BMI, the real question of concern is the proportion of your body that is comprised of fat. With new technology, the amount of fat in your body no longer has to be estimated. It can be known exactly, to the ounce. Although you may want to grimace and groan at the thought that you can determine the proportion of body fat to the ounce, try your best to view this news positively. Knowledge is power, and the goal for you in this chapter is to take control of your body and your weight.

Taking the Guesswork Out of Body Composition

In the recent past, the proportion of "fat" in the body was merely contrasted to the proportion of "nonfat." Some of you may have had fat percentage estimates from skin fold caliper measurements of upper arms or thighs. This inexpensive method of measurement will give you a ballpark guess of your body's fat to nonfat proportions. Unfortunately, it is also not very accurate and usually underestimates actual body fat. The Dual Energy X-Ray Absorptiometry (DEXA) takes the guesswork out of fat measurement.

The DEXA, which is an open scan, just like your bone density scan, can give you an accurate measurement of the fat, bone, and muscle mass in your body. You merely lie down on a completely open table—no needles, no pain, no claustrophobic metal, clanging tunnel. The DEXA scan will yield an overall "picture" (literally) of your body fat, muscle mass, and bone, as well as give a separate measurement analysis for each arm, leg, and the trunk. This procedure (depending on where you go) can be relatively inexpensive—about one hundred dollars at a university center or medical school.

Not surprisingly, a DEXA scan also serves as a bone density assessment. Your insurance might pay for it, or at least a portion of it. An annual DEXA scan can track your increase in muscle or bone mass as you implement your exercise program. Since it yields specific bone, muscle, and fat analysis for different areas of your body, it can give you feedback about specific areas of strength or weakness.

There are also body fat scales on the market for home use that claim to give an accurate reading of body fat percentage. From what I can tell based on consumer guide reviews, the DEXA is by far the most accurate assessment method available. Body fat scales, depending on the quality, are still vulnerable to significant error, but may be more reliable than skin fold measurements. These body fat scales typically work by estimating fat based on impedance of a low-level electrical current through the body from the scale.

So, returning to our 150-pound lady, let's say that she just got her DEXA scan and discovered that she has 36 percent body fat. How does she know exactly what that means?

Age	EXCELLENT 1	VERY GOOD 2	GOOD 3	FAIR 4	POOR 5
19-24	< 19	19.1 - 22	22.1 -25	25.1 - 30	> 30
25-29	< 19	19.1 - 22	22.1 - 25	25.1 -30	> 30
30-34	< 20	20.1 - 23	23.1 - 26	26.1 - 31	> 31
35-39	< 21	21.1 - 24	24.1 - 28	28.1 - 32	> 32
40-44	< 23	23.1 - 26	26.1 - 29	29.1 - 33	> 33
45-49	< 24	24.1 - 27	27.1 - 31	31.1 - 34	> 34
50-54	< 27	27.1 - 31	31.1 - 34	34.1 - 37	> 37
55 +	< 28	28.1 - 31	31.1 -34	34.1 -38	> 38

This would place her in an "average" category of body fat. Next, she should determine her calorie intake and output, and then design a nutritional and exercise program to put her plan into play.

Calories

I like to think of calories as little energy units. The calories in food are energy units used by your body to live and to go about daily activities.

Basal Metabolic Rate

Your basal metabolic rate (BMR) is the amount of energy spent at rest in a neutral environment. BMR is that amount of energy needed to sustain basic life, run your body's vital functioning, and keep you heart, lungs, brain, and other vital organs going.

As you already suspect, BMR decreases with age and loss of lean body mass. This is one of the reasons why we all have a tendency to gain weight as we age. BMR increases with lean muscle mass. This means that the greater the muscle mass, the more calories are burned by just "hanging out." This is why the men in your life can get away with eating more calories. Men usually have more lean muscle mass than women and therefore burn more calories just sitting around than we do.

Unfortunately, cardio fitness (aerobic fitness) does *not* impact BMR directly, but it does affect resting energy calorie consumption, which is good! BMR is affected not only by the proportion of fat to lean muscle, age, and gender, but also by genetics, stress levels, body temperature, the temperature of the environment in which you live, your current weight and body expanse, and the type of exercise you do.

Genetics

You have no control over who your grandparents and parents were. You do have control about how you manage the genes they handed down to you. Some women inherit faster metabolisms than others. Looking at the weight of your ancestors will give you a clue as to what you inherited. Virtually everyone on one side of my family is obese. I used to say that I inherited a "fat gene," but as I became more educated I realized that what I really inherited was a slow basal metabolic rate. From my more informed perspective, I now see this realization as good information. This insight has helped me be more attuned to revving up my BMR.

The thyroid gland also impacts BMR. Higher thyroxin increases BMR; lower thyroxin decreases it. If you have concerns about your BMR, talk to your doctor about your thyroid gland and ensure that it is functioning within normal limits.

Stress Levels

Stress increases your BMR. Obviously, increased stress levels are harmful and you do not want to increase your stress levels in order to burn calories. If you are of normal weight, though, and under extreme stress, know that you might have to provide more fuel for your body under these conditions than you would normally.

Body Temperature

The warmer your body is, the more calories you will burn. Be in tune with your body and don't fight feeling a little heated or sweating when you exercise. If you come from a workout *without* needing a shower, question your level of intensity. Rule of thumb? If you can talk while you exercise, then you probably are not overdoing it.

Environmental Temperature

Just like the temperature inside your body affects BMR, the temperature outside your body affects it, too. Exposure to extreme cold or heat can increase BMR.

Your Weight and Your Expanse

The heavier your weight, the greater your BMR. This is why the two-hundred-pound woman can lose weight faster than her lighter-weight counterpart. Skin surface matters also. A small woman weighing 150 pounds will likely have a lower BMR than a tall woman of the same weight who has more skin expanse.

Exercise

Exercise that builds lean muscle mass while decreasing fat increases your BMR. Muscle and fat cells are like apples and oranges. Once you build muscle, it does *not* turn into fat. Aerobic exercise increases your BMR indirectly. Physical activity in the morning will likely give you a metabolic boost and you will get more bang for your buck than exercise in the evening.

Exercise is a lot more than an hour of purposeful work at the gym. It is walking up the stairs instead of taking the elevator. It is walking around the room while you think or walking to lunch instead of driving. Exercise is anything you do in place of being sedentary.

Obviously many factors affect BMR. Some of these factors are within your control, some are not. It is important to know your BMR so you will know how many calories you can take in per day in order to break even. Many people call this the break-even point, or caloric maintenance. This number will help you set workable and realistic weight-loss goals.

What Is Your BMR?

BMR can be measured, but has to be under somewhat restrictive guidelines. BMR assessment requires a twelve-hour fast and must be conducted while a person is at complete rest. A more common estimate, resting metabolic rate (RMR), is a bit easier to obtain. BMR and RMR are complicated assessments involving gas analysis and either direct or indirect calorimetry, which takes into account your age, gender, height, and weight. Many health clubs and most medical schools can provide this assessment if you want to get this technical. But if you want to keep things simple, just use a guesstimate. Then you can "test drive" your guesstimate and adjust it as needed.

BMR Guesstimate Formula

Use this formula for an adult woman to guesstimate the number of calories you burn just getting through the day.

$$BMR = 655 + (4.3 \times \text{weight in pounds}) + (4.3 \times \text{height in inches}) - (4.7 \times \text{age})$$

Example: 150-pound, 62-inch, 50-year-old woman
$655 + (4.3 \times 150) + (4.3 \times 62) - (4.7 \times 50) = 1{,}331$

Our 150-pound, sixty-two-inch, fifty-year-old sample lady can consume about 1,330 calories daily and break even. If she wanted to lose weight, she would simply need to take in fewer calories or burn more. Ideally, she would do both.

Remember that BMR by this formula is a guesstimate. It will underestimate your break-even calories if you are fit or have a good amount of lean muscle mass. It will overestimate your break-even calories if you are overweight or have a good amount of fat.

Calorie Input

There are a lot of ways to think about calorie intake and output, but I have a personal plan that is nearly foolproof. Calories count, so you have to count calories. When I want to lose weight, I just burn more calories than I consume on a daily basis. I know that if I don't burn all my daily calories, they will end up on my body in an undesirable, unwelcome, and unattractive place. When I am in a maintenance mode (keeping my weight steady), I just consume about what I burn. I am never in a weight-gain mode, but for those of you who are, I begrudgingly advise that you eat more than you burn.

Let's start with the easiest part of the plan: calculating calories burned. Use a calorie book, food packaging information, or any of the many free online programs to calculate caloric value of foods and drinks.

Be smart about calories; learn about them. A nighttime calorie is the same as a morning calorie. A dense calorie is the same caloric unit as a liquid calorie. Consider a fat calorie in this context of weight-loss discussion as the same energy unit as a carbohydrate calorie or a protein calorie. A calorie is a calorie is a calorie when you are thinking exclusively in terms of weight loss. From a nutritional perspective, the type of calorie ingested (fat, carbohydrate, sugar, etc.) is vitally important. Nevertheless, from a sheer weight-loss point of view, all calories are created equal. It's the total number of calories ingested that matters.

Our sample lady could eat 1,330 calories of ice cream or 1,330 calories of broccoli—it does not matter, in terms of losing weight. It does matter in terms of overall health and nutrition. Dr. Sahni, who wrote our nutritional chapter, would rightly advise you to derive calories from the cute, green cruciferous veggie rather than from the sugar- and fat-laden Baskin-Robbins delight. She is thinking big picture: cancer risk, illness risk, and overall health and wellness. Nevertheless, all calories are created equal, so set your goal on ingesting calories from foods that are good for you.

There is only one way to know calorie input: you must record it in some way. A food journal, a daily mental calorie tally, or keeping notes online throughout the day will help you track the calories consumed. Remember that even vitamins and supplements have calories (particularly protein powders and supplements) so remember to count them, too.

I would like to say that I keep mental track of everything I put in my mouth. The truth of the matter is that I do not—I am guilty of a little selective forgetting on occasion. A glass of wine, a cookie here or there, or "tasting" the cottage fries of a friend's meal during lunch—all of these count. I do not know of any way to keep up with calorie input, other than being precise about keeping some sort of record.

Most restaurant and fast-food chains publish information on food and beverage calories. It is more difficult to guesstimate the caloric content of foods served by the charming café on the corner. Although you can try to micro-manage your dining out order by requesting no sauces or lemon juice grilling, the truth of the matter is that when you eat out you cannot know for sure how many calories you are actually taking in. If you are small or are close to your ideal weight range and are trying to shed the last few pounds, a few hundred daily calories can make a difference between gaining and losing weight over a week's time.

Calorie Output

Calculating calorie output is more challenging because it varies greatly from person to person. Calories burned, of course, depend on your BMR. Most people overestimate calories burned and, not surprisingly, underestimate their calorie intake, so it is important to give this equation close attention.

CHOCOLATE IS A MAJOR FOOD GROUP, ISN'T IT?

From the previous section you already have a guesstimate of how many calories you should take in to break even. Trial and error with weekly weighing will help you adjust your allowable break-even caloric intake up or down. Remember that weight can fluctuate by a couple of pounds during the week or even during the day, so it is best to weigh at the same time from day to day. With a little practice, you will develop expertise in predicting how many calories you burn on a daily basis.

The key to perfecting your accuracy in estimating break-even calories burned lies in good record keeping through the scales and a journal. Estimating the calories burned daily is tricky—they will vary greatly depending on your level of activity, or even when you engage in such activity.

If you're like me, your activity level might vary greatly from day to day. Even though I try to exercise every day, I am much more active on weekends when I play outside than I am during the workweek sitting at my desk. My daily burn rate ranges from 1,200 to 2,000 calories depending on how long I sit at my desk. Therefore, I try to match my caloric intake to my activity level to keep my weight balanced. I have a small body frame, so if I miss this calculation by even a few hundred calories, I can gain weight. This happens more often than I would like to admit.

Much like food calorie books, there are also books and online resources that will provide estimates of calories burned by activities ranging from lifting weights to aerobic exercise to horseback riding or golf.[7] You can even find calories burned for vacuuming and dusting. Any and all activity counts.

How Many Calories Do I Have to Burn to Lose Weight?

You have to create a deficit of 3,500 calories to lose a pound. This is why it is so important to know your input and output. Going back to our sample lady: if she burns about 1,330 calories a day, she needs to either cut her calorie consumption by 3,500 calories or increase her caloric burn by that amount in order to lose a pound.

Burning 1,330 daily calories is not much, so she would need to find a way to decrease input as well as increase output. For example, she would need to create a daily deficit of 250 calories in order to lose the pound over a two-week period. She could decide to take in fifty calories less daily and burn an extra two hundred calories daily to reach her goal. Obviously, the winning formula always involves increasing calorie output while at the same time decreasing calorie input. And, if you do not have much weight to lose, it might be the only combination that will work without risking your health.

Keep It Slow and Steady

In order to stay healthy, keep your weight loss slow and steady. The National Institute of Health recommends losing no more than 10 percent of body weight over a six-month period. This fits with our philosophy as well. Set realistic goals and take small steps. Keeping it slow and steady is the best way to lose weight and to keep it off. The exception to slow and steady weight loss would be if you are obese and your health is at high risk. Under these conditions, your physician might well recommend quicker or more invasive weight-loss procedures than we recommend in this book.

Let's return one more time to our example. If our 150-pound lady wants to lose twenty-five pounds in order to improve her health, she would want to lose fifteen pounds over a six-month period, which would put her at 135 pounds. Then she would take her new weight, 135 pounds, calculate her next 10 percent, and lose the last ten pounds over the next four to five months.

Realistically, getting to her target weight will take nearly a year. But progress can begin immediately with a daily deficit of calories. Small steps, losing about two pounds a month, are doable. If she were heavier, she could lose more weight during the six-month period. Trust me on this: it works.

Weigh Every Day

Weigh every morning, right after you finish all your early morning personal business. I do not know a more delicate way to put it. I know there are people out there saying don't weigh every day because you will get discouraged by normal one- to two-pound fluctuations. Ditch that advice. Weigh every morning without fail; it serves many purposes.

Weighing every day will give you inarguable feedback about whether your estimations of calories in and calories out are accurate. You will feel great, moving that number on the scale week by week. Weighing every day keeps you in touch with where you really are and reminds you of your daily goal of input and output, whatever it may be. Finally, research studies indicate that people who weigh every day are more successful in maintaining their desired weight than people who do not.

What Is an Ideal Weight?

This is your decision. The Centers for Disease Control issues normal weight range estimates for gender, age, height, and body frame (the Body Mass Index Table). It is helpful to know these statistics so you can determine your own reference range. As a friend of mine often says, she would be the perfect weight if she were six foot seven. If you find yourself in this position, set a clear goal and start on it today. Tables can guide you to a healthy range, but in the end, determining your ideal weight is your personal decision. Don't be reluctant to think in terms of ideal weight. Your health is at stake, not to mention quality of life and feeling good about yourself.

Remember, a pound of fat weighs sixteen ounces and a pound of muscle weighs sixteen ounces. A pound of fat around your waist will put you in a larger jean size than a pound of muscle around your waist. I have an acquaintance with twin daughters; one is athletic and one is not. Looking at their photos, I cannot tell a difference in size—in fact, they wear the same clothing size. What is amazing, though, is that there is nearly a twenty-five-pound difference in the weights of these two girls. As Martha Stewart would say, "Muscle is a good thing."

Even though losing weight may be your immediate goal, the achievement of health and wellness is truly the plum you seek.

Develop Your Own Plan

There are a million diets out there, but nothing is going to work as well as the plan that you develop to suit your body, goals, and lifestyle. Some of you may find that focusing on caloric burn will be at the heart of your personalized weight-loss plan. Others may find that limiting caloric intake may have higher priority than caloric burn. Some of you may determine to cook at home more and eat out less. Remember that the most successful plans tend to be those that focus on both caloric intake and output.

People are not the same, so it doesn't make sense to think that a particular diet plan will work the same for everyone. Maybe you will want to completely change your diet. Maybe you will want to continue eating the same foods, but eat less. There really is no right and wrong about losing weight if you are cognizant of what goes in your body. It's up to you to determine, even if it is through trial and error, what works best for you. Now that you are armed with the reliable information in this chapter, you are ready to be your own best coach.

Seven-Step Plan

Here's a chart of the steps of weight loss that should make it easy to think about your weight-loss plan.

SEVEN-STEP PLAN: EXAMPLE: 150-pound, 62-inch, 50-year-old woman

STEP ONE Body Mass Index	Weight in Pounds ÷ by height in inches squared x 705 150 ÷ 4,290 x 705 **BMI = 24.7**
STEP TWO BMI Category	Category = Between Ideal & Overweight
STEP THREE Adjust Category based on Body Composition?	Yes – DEXA Scan indicates 36% Body Fat. Determine that real category is "Overweight" rather than "Normal" (See Center for Disease Control & Prevention Chart)
STEP FOUR Determine Total Amount of Weight to Lose	**25 Pounds**
STEP FIVE Weight Loss goal of the next 6 months	10% of Total body Weight = **15 pounds**
STEP SIX Basal Metabolic Rate	BMR = 1331 * * Adjust up or down to compensate for activity level, body composition, etc.
STEP SEVEN Total Calories Per Week to	15 pounds over 6 months = 2.5 pounds/month Needed monthly deficit per month = 8750 calories/month

*At the end of six months, recalculate for the remaining ten pounds to achieve your total goal.

Components of Your Plan

Use the Seven-Step Plan to get your numbers in place.

Keep some sort of record of your calorie intake and output, to ensure the accuracy of the calculations in your plan.

Remember, it takes a 3,500-calorie deficit to shed a pound.

- Your weight-loss goal should be no more than 10 percent of your current weight over a six-month period.

- Keep it slow and steady. Celebrate each small step (but not with dessert!).

- Remain optimistic. You will do what you envision. If you envision success, you will achieve it.

- Design your own plan, taking into account your lifestyle and preferences.

- If the plan doesn't work, go through the troubleshooting ideas presented in the next section.

- Trust the process—it will work.

Troubleshooting: Why Isn't My Plan Working?

If you are following your own plan, you must give it time. Sometimes, drastic changes in your caloric intake and output will throw your body into a "conserving" energy mode. If this happens, it will last only a few weeks. So give your plan a few weeks before you decide it is not working.

If you have followed your plan for thirty days with no result, then you may be battling an unknown organic problem. Run, do not walk, to your doctor's office for advice.

If you are sure your health is good, you have implemented your plan for thirty days, and you're still "stuck" with your weight, then you are either underestimating your caloric intake or overestimating your caloric burn, or both. Should this happen, keep a detailed written food journal and a detailed exercise record. Be meticulous, so you will know your exact caloric intake and output day by day.

Tasha's Story

Tasha's story will inspire you. She started our conversation by telling me that her road to wellness began with a simple decision, but that love from a friend who is "pure of heart" sustained her journey. She said that our interview might take a while because there were no short-term solutions to long-term problems.

Born to an impoverished single mother, Tasha was the fifth girl. She was abandoned at the hospital, even though her mother had two more children, both boys, and kept them. Tasha eventually came to the home of her grandmother, who was unable to give her the protection and care that children deserve.

By the time Tasha was in the fourth grade, she was her grandmother's caretaker. Tasha cooked meals the way she had learned from her grandmother: sausages, lard, oils, butter, and gross overeating were traditions of this home. As if life was not already hard enough, Tasha also became a silent victim of molestation during this time. High blood pressure, diabetes, cardiac disease, and finally cancer took her grandmother's life when Tasha was only eleven. She was then passed off to an aunt who grudgingly took her in.

Not surprisingly, Tasha's weight gain started at about age eleven. Tasha remembers that eating was the only event in her life that felt good. She told me stories about how she wanted to be invisible in high school—that she would not bathe, do her hair, or care what she wore to school in order to be "unnoticed." She made passing marks in school, but Tasha had virtually no friends and no family support. She remembered people telling her she was too big to ride in their car. She said she felt so low that if someone bumped into her in the hallway, she would apologize. By the time she graduated from high school, Tasha was only five feet two inches tall, but weighed more than 250 pounds.

Fearing that she was becoming a diabetic, at age twenty-two and at 286 pounds, Tasha finally went to a doctor. She says she will never forget that day. This doctor, who saw her only once, told her if she did not lose weight soon, she would be forever trapped by it. Tasha said that after she left the office, she began to think of herself as a thin person. She just made a decision that it would have to happen, and that the only question she faced was how to do it.

Tasha, being double-jointed, believed that she could be successful with the bending and stretching demands of yoga. At nearly three hundred pounds, she attended her first yoga class and "found her own peace inside to release bad habits." Tasha attended yoga just once weekly for several months but noticed that she made friends. She tearfully recalled being late to class only to find that the instructor had waited for her before he started. Tasha said that on that day she realized she "mattered."

After eight months and twenty pounds lighter, she started two days each week and then quickly moved to three. The following year she attended class six to seven days a week. Tasha said, "I felt like I had finally found something I was good at."

After shedding the first fifty pounds, Tasha became a vegetarian and began pursuing a degree in creative writing. She continued with yoga for two more years.

Today, Tasha is a size 12. She weighs 180 pounds and has recently started working with a personal trainer. She proudly reported that she outdistanced her peers in her community college physical education class and that she scored in the "exceptional" category on her physical fitness test. Tasha says she still has a way to go, but has no doubt she will achieve her goals. She now describes herself as assertive, fun, and not ashamed of herself, her life, or her journey.

Tasha keeps a food journal and a yoga journal, and calls herself a "National Public Radio junkie." She says she cannot get enough advice on wellness, success, or happiness to satisfy her. She told me that her weight loss was part of a whole package, saying that from the very beginning she knew that her attitude and thoughts were her biggest battle. Tasha says she now lives in the moment.

As we wrapped up our visit, I asked Tasha more about the friend who had helped her. Tasha said she had met a woman in yoga who, when she learned Tasha's story, told her, "I will not leave you; I will always be there as a friend." According to Tasha, this simple statement of commitment inspired and sustained her to make this difficult journey.

Wrap-up

As I said in the beginning of this book, we have compiled these health and wellness guidelines because we want our friends, sisters, mothers, and daughters to have good and healthy lives. We want the people we love to take care of their bodies. Keeping your weight in a healthy range will decrease your risk of serious illness. It will help you feel better and enjoy doing more in life. And last, if not least, living in a healthy weight range will boost your self-esteem. We want you to take care of your body!

PART FOUR

WHAT YOU DON'T KNOW MAY KILL YOU

CHAPTER 9

THE GOOD, THE BAD, AND THE UGLY:
Menopause – The Heat Goes On

Thoughts from Mary Jo:

My husband has always kept our home and our office so cold that you could literally hang meat. Our legal assistants keep those small personal heaters in their offices in the middle of the summer because it is so cold they can't type. People see me in wool in Texas in the middle of August, when the temperature is 105 degrees, and think I'm crazy.

While in China on a trip, Mike's hand was bothering him, so we went to a native doctor in search of some ancient Chinese remedy. The first thing the doctor said through the translator was "too much fire inside." I laughed and said he sure got that right. Mike is my own personal heater.

I tell you all this so that you can understand my next story. I remember the day like it was yesterday. I was sitting in a meeting of about thirty lawyers and legal assistants (our weekly Tuesday 7:30 a.m. meeting). All the women had on sweaters or other clothing to keep them warm, and I turned to my husband and said, "Is it hot in here?" It was so quiet in the room that you could have heard a pin drop. Everyone was looking at me like I had grown horns, or at least flipped out. When my husband said, "It is actually quite comfortable," it dawned on me what must have happened. *How can this be?* I thought. *I'm only in my early forties!* And yet it was happening to me, and the heat has gone on for the better part of a decade now.

One of the more bothersome things about hot flashes is that they may occur when you least expect them. My personal favorite happened in the courtroom. My opposing counsel looked over at me, saw me sweating, and really thought he had me on the ropes. It actually turned out to my advantage, because he made a snide remark to the fifty-something female judge and she knew exactly what was going on, since she was experiencing it herself. It gave the judge and me an instant bond.

Gone are the days when the male judge and the male attorney go into the judge's chambers and discuss their hunting trip or the last football game. We took a break, and both lawyers and the judge went into her chambers and discussed how inconvenient hot flashes are. Taught that guy not to make snide remarks!

Over the years, as menopause has no longer been a forbidden topic to discuss in polite company, I have learned to take most of it in stride. When people see me fanning myself on a cold winter day, I simply say, "I am having my own personal summer moment." While I have learned to deal with the embarrassment of the situation, other symptoms of menopause have been far more bothersome.

I am one of those women Dr. Sahni will talk about who has the pleasure of having hot flashes and night sweats. I tried the natural herbal route for several years, taking herbal remedies with some success, but the older I get, the less effective those remedies are. I went to my gynecologist, who explained to me the risks of hormone replacement therapy, but said that ultimately it is a matter of quality of life. I chose quality of life. He put me on a low-dosage patch that I had to change only once a week. The problem was that I started having periods again. Not very heavy, but instead of once a month, it was every day. Egad! I exchanged one problem for another.

After suffering through that ordeal for the better part of the year, I returned to the herbal route. That actually worked pretty well for a few months, and then slowly but surely the hot flashes and night sweats returned with a vengeance, and with two more elements added. My sleep, for the first time in my life, became erratic, which made me grouchy and very tired during the day. I am sure that my staff probably took bets on which monster would come in each day. Would I show up as Barney, or would I show up as a werewolf? But even more troublesome (as if that were not enough) was when it began to be painful to have intercourse. It not only was very painful for me, but for my husband as well. There was not enough Astroglide in the world to make it OK. *Wow, the doctor never told me about this!* This was no longer a "quality of life" issue, but a "this is going to hurt my marriage if I can't have sex with my husband" issue. (I told you that he is very hot-blooded, and that affects him in many ways!)

So, what's a girl to do? It was Dr. Sahni to the rescue! She gave me a simple blood test and determined which hormones were low. All of mine were nonexistent. Dr. Sahni then put me on bio-identical hormones of estradiol, estriol, progesterone, DHEA, and testosterone. Estradiol and estriol are identical to the hormones produced in significant quantities in the human body, primarily by the ovaries. Estrogens are responsible for the development and maintenance of the female reproductive system, secondary sex characteristics, favorable effects on blood cholesterol and lipid profiles, and slowing the progression of osteoporosis, as well as causing proliferation of the endometrium. It is not something that is made by any pharmaceutical company—it is mixed by the pharmacy to meet my specific needs. I take it every night before I go to bed. It is put under the tongue and is absorbed in the body more rapidly that way.

I am happy to report that my hot flashes and night sweats have decreased dramatically and I now sleep like a baby. Just as important, my libido has returned and I can have intercourse without the pain.

Obviously, not all women have the symptoms I experienced, nor do they always last a decade. I certainly hope for your sake that you don't have my experience. Every woman is different, and that is why what you choose to do must be tailor-made for you. If your doctor doesn't understand that, then change doctors. Many women can go to the health food store and get supplements and be very comfortable. Many women have a history of breast cancer in their family and do not want to increase their risk, so they do not want to use hormone replacement therapy. There is no cookie-cutter approach. Educate yourself about menopause and don't be afraid to talk to your friends about their experience and what works for them. Your fifties are a great time in your life! Don't miss them because you are too embarrassed to get help. Let the beat go on—not the heat.

THE GOOD, THE BAD, AND THE UGLY: Menopause – The Heat Goes On

What the Doctor Has to Say: Jyotsna Sahni, M.D.

Few topics cause more confusion than menopause. Even though it's a normal, natural process that happens to all women sooner or later, it seems to be shrouded in mystery and myth. This chapter will help to sort it all out, from the perspective of a woman doctor who's seen hundreds of patients in its throes. To start, it is common and getting more so.

An estimated forty-three million women will go into menopause in the next two decades. And these baby boomers will not take it lying down! There is more research, more studies, and more choices for women today than at any other time in history. It is a great time to be a woman!

Four Main Hormones

There are four main female hormones you ought to know a little about.

Estrogen

The first is estrogen. Actually, there are several estrogens: estrone, estradiol, and estriol, and many others. I put the most stock in estradiol because it's the most powerful and plentiful estrogen before menopause. It gets produced by the ovary and also is produced when others estrogens are converted to it in the bloodstream. A decline in estrogen causes many of the symptoms we associate with menopause, but more about those later.

Progesterone

Progesterone is also made by the ovary; it prepares the uterus for a fertilized egg. It's often called the "pregnancy" hormone. A decline in progesterone also causes symptoms of menopause.

Testosterone

Testosterone is often thought to be a male hormone, but women make it too, in the ovaries. Its decline may also cause a variety of symptoms.

Follicle Stimulating Hormone

Follicle stimulating hormone (FSH) is produced by the pituitary gland in the brain. Its main function is to stimulate the ovary to produce estrogen to prepare eggs for release. I measure it for two purposes. The first is to answer the question, "Can I still get pregnant?" The FSH is the first hormone that fertility doctors check to see if a woman is still able to have a child. The second use is to get a sense of how close a woman is to menopause. The higher the number, the louder the brain is yelling at the ovaries to make more estrogen. The higher the number, the closer she is to menopause and the farther away from having children. Like the other three hormones, FSH can fluctuate, but it tends to change less on a day-to-day basis.

Putting It All Together

To understand the hormonal changes in menopause, you first have to know what happens before menopause. When women are having their periods on a regular basis, they are considered "premenopausal," meaning "before menopause." Typically, this is from when a young girl gets her first period at around twelve years old to her mid-forties. Hopefully she gets her period each month, except when she is pregnant. During this time, estrogen goes up and down like a mountain, peaking at mid-cycle when she's ovulating or releasing an egg. Estrogen builds her uterine lining so that it's a thick, juicy nest for a baby. If the egg doesn't get fertilized, her estrogen and progesterone will drop and she'll shed her uterine lining (get her period), and the whole process will start again the next month.

Before Menopause

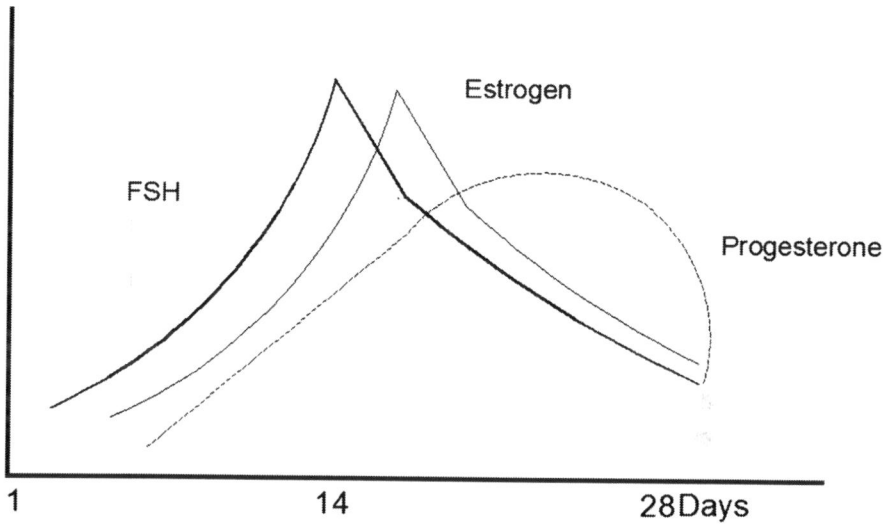

What Is Perimenopause?

The term "perimenopause" refers to the time "around" menopause. It is defined by being forty-five years old and a woman. This is a very arbitrary definition. A better definition might be "intermittent ovarian function." Now her estrogen levels still go up and down over the course of the month, but instead of looking like a mountain, they look more like a rollercoaster ride. Progesterone tends to be low and flat at this time. What this means is that some months everything works properly, in an orderly fashion, the way it should. The woman gets her period when she expects it. Some months are not so predictable. Some women skip their period for two or three months, and then have a heavy bleed. Other women have two or three periods in the same month. Either way, it's hard to handle. Along with irregular periods, many symptoms are likely to occur.

Peri-Menopause

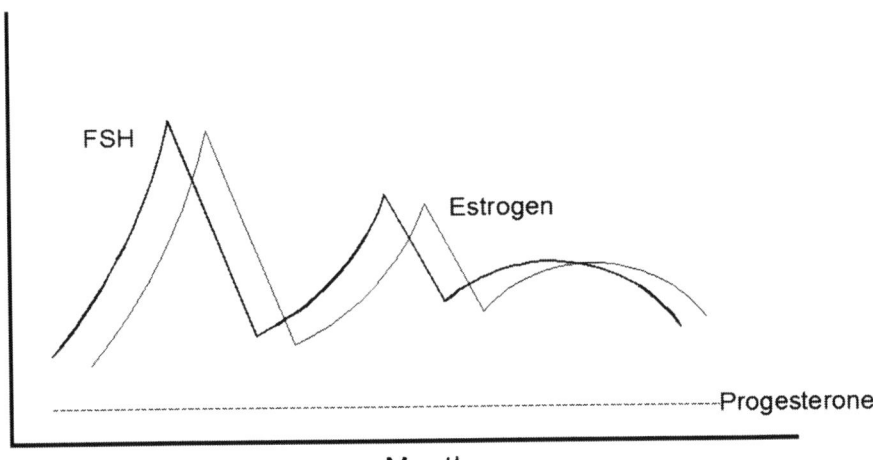

What Is Menopause?

Menopause is defined as having no period for one year. At this time, estrogen and progesterone levels are both low and flat. The ovaries are in the Bahamas sipping on margaritas; they are in retirement and no longer do much work. Occasionally, a woman simply stops having periods and that's the end of the discussion. Most women, however, have some symptoms and feelings about the whole process. The average age of menopause is fifty-one years old, but it can happen earlier or later. About 8 percent of women have menopause before the age of forty. Most women experience menopause within two years of the age their mother did. Sometimes we speed up that process. For example, a total hysterectomy, where a woman has both her ovaries and uterus removed, propels a woman into a sudden "surgical" menopause. Having a tubal ligation for birth control, chemotherapy, or a partial hysterectomy (just the uterus removed) can also lead to an earlier menopause.

After Menopause

```
|                                    ———— FSH




|
|                                    ———— Estrogen
|------------------------------------ ---- Progesterone
|_____
           Months
```

Symptoms of Menopause

Hot Flashes

The classic symptom of menopause is, of course, the hot flash. It's kind of a unique symptom; maybe you get a fever when you get the flu, but not much other than menopause can cause a sudden rise in body temperature. It can happen every hour, every day, or just once a month. Some hot flashes are mild (often called "hot flushes") and pass quickly; others are severe, uncomfortable, and embarrassing. Some women have triggers for hot flashes, such as red wine, spicy foods, or a strong emotion that brings on a blush, which then turns into a hot flash.

It makes sense to avoid triggers if you have them (and to dress in layers at all times!). Hot flashes that occur at night are referred to as night sweats. Some women just kick off the covers because they're a little warm at night; others get up and change their nightgowns and sheets because they've made a puddle in their beds! Some women have either hot flashes or night sweats, some women have both, some have neither.

Some common trigger foods for hot flashes are: caffeine, chocolate, garlic, ginger, cayenne pepper, onions, spicy foods, hot beverages, salty foods, alcohol, and high-fat or acidic foods.

Sleep Disturbance

Another common symptom of menopause is sleep disturbance. The classic menopausal sleep disturbance is this: falling asleep easily at night, but waking up every hour and a half after that. This annoying sleep disturbance is often accompanied by hot flashes and night sweats. In addition to sleep "maintenance" insomnia, women in menopause may also develop "sleep-disordered breathing." The lack of estrogen may make snoring worse and make sleep much less restful.

Finally, the role of estrogen is important in the development of fibromyalgia and depression, which often go hand in hand. Both conditions are associated with a sleep disturbance and occur more often in women than men. Both are common in menopausal women. But the bottom line is this: if you wake up four or five times during the night but fall right back to sleep and it doesn't get in the way of your quality and quantity of sleep, I'm not too worried. On the other hand, if your sleep problem is leaving you tired and irritable the next day, I do worry. Now it's affecting your health. We'll talk more about the importance of sleep later in chapter 13, but for now I'll simply say that good sleep is vital to good health.

Memory Loss

Memory loss is another annoying symptom of menopause. Women tell me every day that they're afraid they're developing premature Alzheimer's disease. When I ask what they can't remember, they tell me names, places, and things. Perhaps they have to make lists of their lists, or line up things in front of the door so they remember them on their way out of the house first thing in the morning. Women also complain of "tip of the tongue" episodes when they can't think of a word but know they know it. There's an area of the brain known as the hippocampus where we make our short-term memories and it's full of estrogen receptors. When in perimenopause and menopause, levels of estrogen plummet and short-term memory suffers. This can be a terribly frustrating symptom of menopause, but take heart. It's often worse early in menopause and better later, when hormones fluctuate less.

Headaches

Headaches are another classic sign of menopause. In fact, over their lifetimes, women typically have two or three times as many headaches as men—not in childhood or in old age, but in the reproductive years when hormone levels change with the menstrual cycle. Fluctuating levels of hormones are the trigger for headaches in many women. This is often seen in premenstrual women. They may get a "period" headache for a day or two before their periods that abates when they actually start to bleed. The same is true in perimenopausal women; when their hormone levels fluctuate they get headaches. These headaches often throb and pound and are untouched by the usual over-the-counter medications. Interestingly, many women with migraines enjoy menopause, because hormone levels are low and migraines may disappear or at least lessen.

Mood Changes

Mood changes are also common at menopause. Let's face it: as women, our hormones do affect our moods. Women become clinically depressed about two or three times more than men over the course of their lifetimes and are especially vulnerable to depression at times of hormonal flux. We clearly see this in premenstrual syndrome and also as postpartum depression. Menopause is no exception. As estrogen levels fluctuate and eventually fall, so may levels of serotonin in the brain. Serotonin is the neurotransmitter that is associated with happy feelings. For example, Prozac works on serotonin receptors. There are savvy psychiatrists today who actually look to estrogen before Prozac in women who are depressed in menopause. Along with depression, feelings of irritability, anxiety, and emotional fragility are common. Sappy TV commercials can suddenly take on grave meaning and bring on tears. Some women describe this fragile mood as a severe case of PMS.

Vaginal Dryness

Dry skin, dry hair, dry eyes, and even vaginal dryness occur at menopause. The first three can be dealt with using various moisturizers, but vaginal dryness is more difficult. It usually begins just with lack of or lessened lubrication during sex play. If that's the only issue, using over-the-counter sexual lubricants often helps. A woman has to get over her fear of the condom aisle at the drugstore because this is where the sexual lubricants are kept. They all taste different, feel different, and smell different, but generally they're cheap and available. I tell women if they don't like one to simply toss it and try another. Put a little on you and your partner and things will slide better. Some brands include Astroglide, Slippery Stuff, and Probe (these were obviously named by men!). Sometimes a woman has dryness not only during sex but the rest of the time, too. There are vaginal moisturizers for this purpose such as Lubrin, Moist Again, and Replens (these were probably named by women!). Again, these are cheap and available over the counter and are worth trying out.

Finally, some women have such severe dryness that more aggressive measures are necessary. When I do pelvic exams on women in my practice, I want to see a pink, moist, juicy vagina. If I see dryness, cracks, or fissures, or hear about frequent yeast and urinary tract infections, or if the speculum hurts too much, then I introduce the idea of using a vaginal estrogen. This is a prescription product, but I tend to hand out these prescriptions quite liberally because they are so safe and effective. Women can use them in conjunction with systemic hormone replacement therapy (such as pills or patches) or alone if vaginal dryness is the only symptom. They are not powerful enough to help with hot flashes, night sweats, sleep disturbance, etc., but they work well for vaginal dryness. Many of the annoying symptoms of menopause simply fade away with time, but vaginal dryness tends to be progressive. Generally, I don't see sixty-five-year-old women with unbearable hot flashes, but almost every sixty-five-year-old woman I see has vaginal dryness.

I prescribe three main products. The first is Estrace cream, a bio-identical estradiol cream that is shot up in the vagina twice a week before bed. It's a little messy but works really well.

The next is Vagifem. It too is estradiol, but in a little pill that is placed at the end of an applicator smaller than a pen and also shot up in the vagina twice a week before bed. It's much less messy than using a cream and it also works very well.

The third product is quite clever; it's a soft plastic ring that's been impregnated with estrogen. The patient places it high in the vagina like a diaphragm and it slowly leaches out estrogen over the course of three months. It's definitely low maintenance, needing to be changed only four times a year. You don't feel it, and neither should anyone else.

These products can be used alone or in conjunction with systemic hormone replacement therapy in the form of pills, patches, creams, etc.

Hormones and Breast Cancer Risk

Women with a history of breast cancer or a fear about it often ask me about the safety of vaginal estrogens. The good news is that many oncologists—cancer doctors—give the green light with regard to this issue. The first reason is that these products contain such a small amount of hormone that it doesn't get absorbed systemically (through the system of the body). This is why these products are no good for hot flashes or night sweats—they are designed to help with vaginal dryness and that's pretty much all they do. By giving estrogen back to the vaginal tissues, you make your own lubrication, prevent or treat atrophy or thinning of the tissues and maintain elasticity, and keep the pH of the vagina in a good range to prevent yeast and other infections.

The other reason cancer doctors allow vaginal estrogen is quality of life. Women taking Tamoxifen for breast cancer tend to be especially plagued by dryness because the drug's job is to block up every drop of estrogen in the body, thereby making vaginal dryness even worse. Again, vaginal estrogens tend to be both safe and effective.

Urinary Symptoms

I also hear about urinary symptoms. Women tell me that they have urinary urgency, frequency, and sometimes incontinence. There are basically two types of incontinence that I see. The first is "stress" incontinence; she leaks urine when she laughs, sneezes, or coughs. She definitely needs to empty her bladder before jumping rope or taking a trampoline class at the health club. Having had children (especially lots of big ones), carrying extra weight, having flabby abdominal and pelvic muscles, and a lack of estrogen in the vagina and surrounding structures are often to blame.

Some women say their incontinence is a strong urge to use the restroom and they simply can't make it in time. This is known as "urge" incontinence.

When women suffer from both of these together, it's known as "mixed" incontinence. There are effective treatments for most incontinence, so it's definitely worth speaking to your doctor about. Addressing the root causes of stress incontinence, using behavioral techniques to suppress the "urge", and/or taking certain medications will usually improve this problem.

Heart Palpitations

Because estrogen modulates the release of adrenaline, women can find themselves with episodes of palpitations or rapid heartbeat. This symptom can be downright scary, and can make a woman fear she's having a heart problem or heart attack. If she's seen in an emergency room or at the doctor's office, she may be told that she's having a panic attack or that the problem is in her head, when in fact it is real. Some physicians are unaware of the role of estrogen in the sympathetic nervous system. Since the sympathetic nervous system governs the "fight or flight" response, when it's kicked up a woman may experience a racing heartbeat, fast breathing, feelings of anxiety, or have a sense of impending doom.

Putting your hormone levels back into balance by using supplements or hormone replacement therapy can be helpful. Avoiding caffeine or other stimulants is a good idea too. An appropriate exercise program, healthy food, adequate rest, and yogic breathing (as described in other chapters) may be necessary to modulate this uncomfortable symptom.

Weight Gain

Women also describe symptoms of testosterone deficiency. Women make testosterone in our ovaries, but we make only about 10 percent of what men do. At menopause, levels of testosterone can decline or even be absent if a woman has lost her ovaries to surgery. Some women may lose lean muscle mass with loss of testosterone. This can slow the body's metabolic rate. Every week it seems an exasperated fifty-one-year old woman storms into my office, telling me that she's eating the same and exercising the same but has gained this stupid five to fifteen pounds, especially around her waist, hips, and thighs. She looks more "rectangular" rather than "hourglass" shaped. She complains that it's not fair and must be her hormones. It is her hormones, but just not the ones she thinks—it is testosterone. So, what does that say about exercise as we grow older? That's right! More of it, and specifically weight training. Lifting weights or doing resistance work allows us to maintain the muscle we've got, or, if we're lucky enough, to make more of it. Muscle mass is what's burning calories as you're sitting here reading this book. Lu Jurcova Phillips and Mary Jo explore in more detail the right exercise programs in chapters 4, 5, and 6.

Thinning Hair

I often suspect low levels of testosterone when a woman tells me that she no longer has to shave her legs or underarms as frequently, or that her pubic hair is thinning out. Thinning body hair is a sign of testosterone loss. Some women lose a lot of hair from their heads around menopause, but this is a different situation. This phenomenon is known as "post-menopausal alopecia" and actually is a result of decreased estrogen, not testosterone. Rogaine for Women, certain supplements, and an appointment with a good dermatologist may be warranted.

Decline in Sexual Interest

Many women experience a decline in sexual interest around menopause. Sexuality is a tremendously complex issue in women and is beyond the scope of this book. Briefly, though, sex drive is both biological and, of course, psychological. Having said that, if you recall the sexual response cycle by Masters and Johnson, there are four stages: The first is arousal, followed by plateau, orgasm, and recovery. Arousal ("Hi, I'm turned on!") is governed by testosterone, the biologic trigger for libido. Without it, sex drive is typically low. But as I joke with my patients, if you hate your husband it doesn't matter how much testosterone you have, you're not going to want to make love to him.

Women are much more than a sum of their hormones. The psychological aspects are equally as important as the biological; relationship issues, body image, aging issues, childhood trauma, and societal messages about sex all can have potent effects on sexual desire. A counselor, nurse, or doctor trained in women's sexuality can help navigate these complex issues.

As a women's physician, I do check levels of testosterone. If the story fits the numbers, I may supplement with natural bio-identical testosterone at times. For many women with low testosterone levels and low libido, replacement is very helpful. While I can't make a woman twenty-two years old again, often I can help her feel more like her old self. This is especially true if a woman has lost her ovaries to surgery. Since the ovaries are the largest source of testosterone in a woman's body, hysterectomy can sometimes be devastating to sexual functioning.

Treatment with too much testosterone can also be devastating—acne, hair growth, and aggression are never fun. Refusing to ask directions at a gas station when you're lost is, of course, another sign of too much testosterone. If I end up giving a woman too much, we simply stop the dose for about a week, let the hormone degrade in the system, and start again with a smaller dose. I monitor patients by seeing how they feel and also by lab testing.

Low Energy Level

Testosterone may also govern energy levels and an overall sense of well-being. Energy is hard to quantify, but if you think of the typical eighteen-year-old boy, he's got big muscles, lots of sex drive, has to shave his face twice a day, and is full of energy. Some women with testosterone deficiency complain of fatigue. Of course, sleep deprivation can also add to fatigue. The role of testosterone often goes unrecognized as an important part in the quality of the lives of some women.

Higher Cholesterol

Other changes that occur in menopause are less obvious. These may include worsening cholesterol values. For example, LDL (or "the lousy, loser" cholesterol) tends to increase by about 10 to 15 percent in women in menopause. The "healthy, happy" cholesterol, or HDL, tends to drop by about 10 to 15 percent. Both go in the wrong direction and may put a woman at higher risk for clogged arteries, leading to heart disease. Along with weight control, healthy eating with attention paid to decreasing saturated fats helps control LDL values. Regular exercise may help boost both HDL values and fitness levels.

Loss of Bone Density

Another less obvious change that occurs with loss of estrogen at menopause is the loss of bone density. This may lead to osteopenia ("thinning bone") and osteoporosis ("porous bone"). When it comes to bone loss, menopause is the most vulnerable time in a woman's life. Unfortunately, the first symptom of osteoporosis is a broken bone. By then, it's too late. It makes me both mad and sad when I see a little old lady all bent over, because osteoporosis is both a preventable and treatable disease. More about this in the following chapter.

Hormones: To Take or Not to Take

Every week I give a lecture on menopause, and every week I say what I'm going to say to you now: I don't put all women on hormones and I don't keep all women off hormones. Ultimately it's your decision—based on your fears, your needs, your family history, and other risk factors. It's your decision because at the end of day, it's your body. Like I said earlier, there is more information, more research, and more choices than ever before regarding hormones. It really is a good time to be a woman.

As a physician, I know I can help your hot flashes, night sweats, sleep disturbance, memory loss, mood changes, headaches, and vaginal dryness by giving you hormones. Clearly hormone treatments are effective for many of the symptoms of menopause, but I'm not anxious to give all women hormones at all times. One thing I worry about is breast cancer.

THE GOOD, THE BAD, AND THE UGLY: Menopause – The Heat Goes On

Breast cancer is common and scary. Dr. Kristi McIntyre will talk in detail about breast cancer in chapter 12. She is an oncologist and an expert on breast cancer. I tend to deal with women who don't have breast cancer but who (like all women) may be at risk for it. I have to do my best to make decisions about a woman's risk for breast cancer before I consider giving her hormones.

One traditional method we have to predict who will get breast cancer is the Gail Model of Breast Cancer Assessment. Basically, it's a statistical computer program designed by the National Cancer Institute that asks you a series of questions and assesses your five-year risk and your lifetime risk of breast cancer. The first question is "What's your age?" The older you are, the more likely you are to get breast cancer. This is because you have outlived other diseases that could have killed you at a younger age. After being a woman, age is the most important risk factor for breast cancer. (One percent of breast cancers do occur in men.) While we're talking about ages, how old were you when you had your first child? If you never had children, or had your first child after the age of thirty, it does increase your risk for breast cancer a small amount. The earlier you started your family, the more children you had, and the more you breast-fed, the better it is for your breasts. This is a bit of a dilemma for young women today who are typically having smaller families later or choosing not to have children at all.

Family History

We also ask about family history of breast cancer. The concern is about close family—first-degree relatives. This means mothers and sisters. Second cousins twice removed are too far from your genes to have any bearing on your risks. If you tell me that your mother had breast cancer, my next question will be, "How old was she when she was diagnosed?" If she was eighty-five, I'm not going to bat an eye. On the other hand, if you tell me forty-five, I'll raise a concerned eyebrow. It seems that the younger the breast cancer, and especially if before menopause, the more aggressive and more genetic it is.

Biopsies and Abnormal Mammograms

We also ask about number of breast biopsies and abnormal mammograms. Let's face it: today if there's even a smudge on the mammogram, they take a bite of breast tissue and look at it under the microscope. If everything is normal ("benign"), I won't worry about it. But if there are changes that aren't quite normal but not quite cancer either, I'll put that into my analysis.

Exposure to Estrogen

Finally we ask about exposure to estrogen. How old were you when you got your first period? Your first period is really your first real exposure to estrogen. You could have been eleven years old when you started menstruating; eleven is considered perfectly normal. Sixteen is considered normal, too. But the five-year difference puts the eleven-year-old at higher risk for breast cancer because she's had five more years of estrogen exposure stimulating her breasts and possibly making mistakes in that cell stimulation. Mistakes in cells also can be called cancerous changes.

We can't do too much about when we start our periods. However, we often do affect when we stop our periods—with surgery and so on. I love to tell the story of two women who saw me back-to-back on a Thursday afternoon. One was a thirty-seven-year-old who had had a total hysterectomy and was thrilled to be done with her periods. The next woman was a fifty-seven-year-old who came in, stomped her foot, and told me that she was still having a regular period each month. She said that none of her friends were still having theirs and demanded, "What's wrong with me?" I asked her when her mother had gone through menopause. She pulled out her cell phone right there in my office, speed-dialed her mother in Boca Raton, and proceeded to have a conversation. Within minutes, she had my answer. "Sixty," she said. Sixty! I tried to reassure her that nothing was wrong; that she was simply way on the extreme side of the bell curve for age of menopause.

One year later, she came to visit and proudly announced she was finally in menopause. I said, "Congratulations! I knew it would happen sooner or later!" The difference between these two women is not just twenty more years of periods, but twenty more years of estrogen exposure to the breasts. More estrogen exposure may mean more risk for cancer.

What about birth control pills? After all, they're hormones, too. Well, the good news is that no study shows that birth control pills increase risk of breast cancer in women at *average* risk for breast cancer. Also, studies do show that women who have been on the pill for five years or more cumulatively over the course of their lifetimes actually cut their risk of ovarian cancer by about 50 percent! They also cut their risk for uterine cancer, but that protection seems to last just while taking the pill, while the ovarian cancer protection seems to be lifelong. I guess these hormones can't be all bad.

The big controversy about the use of hormones really lies after menopause. The Women's Health Initiative (WHI) was the largest study of its sort to look at the effects of hormones on postmenopausal women. It got a lot of press when the study was halted prematurely in July 2002 because of some scary results. What was seen in the study was a 26 percent increase in incidence of breast cancer in women taking Prempro for more than five years. The media took this story and ran with it, and women all over America were confused and frightened. Many women stopped taking their hormones cold turkey. My office phone rang off the hook for days on end. But the statistics were tricky and hard to follow. We were told by the media that there was a 26 percent increase in the risk of breast cancer. But in fact that is really a very small change.

To make the statistics simpler to understand, think of it this way: what we know now is that of ten thousand women not on hormone replacement therapy, thirty get breast cancer. If they do take hormones, thirty-eight women in ten thousand would get breast cancer. In both cases, about 3/100th of one percent of women will get breast cancer. I totally agree that thirty-eight is a larger number than thirty, but what is the difference between thirty and thirty-eight? It is 26 percent. This does not mean that 26 percent of all women taking hormones will get breast cancer, but what the change would be from baseline. This increase didn't actually make "statistical significance," which is like throwing darts at the wall and seeing what side they fall on. Do they fall on the cancer side because hormones cause cancer, or do they fall on that side because that group of women just happened to get more cancer by chance? The study was stopped before its scheduled end because the scientists did not want to put women at increased risk, but it turns out breast cancer wasn't what prompted them to stop the study. However, that's all the news media seemed to report. Nonetheless, this concern about more cancer with hormones had been raised in other studies before and it's certainly something to consider.

Heart Attacks and Strokes

The real reason the WHI was stopped was an increase in heart attacks and strokes. This was a total shock to cardiologists everywhere who for the previous twenty years had been pushing hormones to prevent heart disease. One reason for this may simply have been the fact that the average age of women in this study was sixty-four, a little older and more at risk for heart attacks and strokes than younger women. The other concern was centered on the forms of hormones used in the study. Prempro, the study drug, is a combination of Premarin and Provera. As I detail in the next section, Provera, a powerful, synthetic progestagin, may elevate cholesterol and blood pressure and cause spasm of blood vessels, which may then have led to more heart attacks and strokes. Interestingly, if women do have a heart attack or stroke while taking Prempro, they usually do it early on, within the first year or so. If they do fine on hormones during the first year or two, usually by years four and five they actually are healthier than women not taking hormones at all.

THE GOOD, THE BAD, AND THE UGLY: Menopause – The Heat Goes On

There were actually two arms to the Prempro study: one involved Prempro itself and the other one involved Premarin only (for women who had had hysterectomies and didn't need Provera). Strangely, the women taking Premarin alone did not have more heart attacks, nor did they have more breast cancer than women not taking hormones at all. They did have more strokes, which was not too surprising because we've known for a long time that estrogen can increase clotting risk. (This is why women over the age of thirty-five who smoke have been discouraged from using birth control pills.) But synthetic progestagins do have their risks as well. Looking at this data, many doctors pointed to the Provera, *not the estrogen*, as the bad actor. I know this hormone story is totally confusing, but this is why doctors have to be really careful in prescribing these powerful drugs; they can heal and they can harm.

How Do I Treat the Symptoms of Menopause?

Soy

I think it's always good to try the simpler, gentler approach to treating menopausal symptoms, because some women only need a little help and the over-the-counter products may be effective enough. Herbs like black cohosh, red clover, and phytoestrogens from soy may be helpful. Soy is a "phytoestrogen," or estrogen-like plant compound; it provides isoflavones known as genestein and diadzein. In some studies, these have been shown to decrease the risk of heart disease and cancer, promote bone health, and help with hot flashes and other menopausal symptoms. Soy should be gotten from food sources like tofu, tempeh, soy milk, or edamame in as clean a source as possible.

Unfortunately, most soy in the United States has been genetically modified to withstand high levels of pesticide use. Look for "non-GMO" (non-genetically modified) or "organic" on labels. It's best to avoid "soy protein concentrate," which may contain more soy than anyone could possibly get from diet alone. Instead, look for the terms soy protein, soy protein isolate, or textured soy protein. Consider substituting tofu for mozzarella cheese in pizza recipes and for ricotta cheese in lasagna, using soy milk in lattes or cappuccinos, and using soy flour instead of wheat flour in breads, rolls, pancakes, and muffins.

There's a controversy about soy in the medical and nutritional literature; some say it prevents breast cancer, some say it causes breast cancer. Both may be true. Proponents of soy often cite studies done in Japan, where the population has a low incidence of breast cancer and high consumption of soy in the diet. It's also true that the women in Japan have different genetics than the average American woman, weigh less, and consume less alcohol and red meat (other possible contributors to breast cancer). I say that in a healthy, varied diet, soy is a good thing, but I ask my patients with breast cancer to avoid it. As an added benefit, 25 g of soy protein daily may decrease cholesterol!

Flaxseeds

Flaxseeds are a healthy food for women for three reasons. Ground flaxseed (or flaxseed oil) provides a compound known as lignans, which in some studies has been shown to prevent breast cancer in women. The seeds themselves also contain fiber for elimination (I cure constipation with flaxseeds all the time; unlike Metamucil or Citrucel, flax has additional healthy properties). Finally, the flaxseeds contain a healthy omega-3 fat known as alpha linolenic acid. Flaxseeds have a mild, nutty flavor; they can be sprinkled on salad, fruit, or oatmeal, and are a healthy addition to a good diet.

What Is the Best Hormone Replacement for Me?

There are a lot of estrogen products on the market. Some are synthetic; some are "bio-identical." Bio-identical products are considered to be more natural, looking like the hormones we make ourselves in our ovaries. Often they are derived from soybeans, prepared in a lab, and prescribed by a doctor. Some are sold at large chain drugstores and manufactured by large pharmaceutical houses, some are prepared in small compounding pharmacies, and others are sold over the counter as supplements.

Typically, over-the-counter products are safe, partly because they simply don't have many active ingredients. While they may not hurt you, they may not help you either.

Premarin – Last Choice

If I had to prescribe an estrogen, Premarin would be my last choice. It was all we had for a long time, but now we have better choices. Premarin stands for "pregnant mare's urine." First of all, that's a gross idea. But I'm a doctor and gross doesn't bother me too much. Second, there are six or seven equine (horse) estrogens in Premarin, none of which mimics what the human ovary makes. Third, and very importantly, Premarin has been shown in some small studies to break down preferentially into a toxic metabolite (4-OH estrone) associated with breast cancer. I think we have better choices and should use them.

Estradiol

If I had to prescribe estrogen in a pill, I would go with estradiol. It is bio-identical, sold at your neighborhood pharmacy, and usually covered by prescription plans. But when you swallow a pill, it goes into the stomach, is digested, and is sent to the liver for detoxification. The liver has many jobs. It makes cholesterol and clotting factors, and it detoxifies medications like Lipitor and estrogen, along with chardonnay and pesticides. When you take an oral estrogen, you end up needing a bigger dose, and you may increase your triglycerides and clotting risks.

First Choice

If I had my first choice, I'd give you estrogen through your skin (transdermal). A patch like Climara or Vivelle is a good choice.

By being absorbed through the skin, patches bypass the liver, and often you can get away with a smaller dose and worry less about cholesterol and clotting effects. Also, they provide a slow, even absorption of estrogen over the course of the week. This means fewer estrogen level highs and lows, and hopefully fewer triggers for mood changes in women prone to depression, anxiety, and panic attacks. Also, patches provide fewer triggers in women who are prone to migraines and other headaches. In addition, patches come in numerous doses. That's nice because I don't want to give you too little or too much hormone. If you go to the trouble of taking hormones and still have hot flashes, night sweats, etc., to me it seems pointless to be taking them in the first place. On the other hand, these drugs may have serious consequences, so I don't want you to take one drop more than you actually need.

Cream or Gel

In addition to patches, there is a nice emollient cream of estrogen known as Estrasorb that you rub into your thighs each day. They also make Estrogel, a gel that is similar. Being a bit of a control-freak doctor, I'm a little reluctant to prescribe these because I don't always know exactly how much you are using or how well they absorb in the skin of different people. But both of these products are estradiol and overall probably are good choices.

Plastic Ring

There is also Femring, a soft plastic ring that is inserted in the vagina and lasts for three months. The difference is that it has enough hormones to help not only vaginal dryness, but also the systemic symptoms of menopause like hot flashes. Again, this is estradiol, but in a very clever, convenient form.

Compound

Sometimes I compound estradiol with estriol and other hormones at my local compounding pharmacy. I can put several different hormones together at very precise doses. I can increase or decrease those doses based upon what my patient needs. I usually ask the pharmacy to make a lozenge to suck on, but sometimes we make a cream. Not all compounding pharmacies are good and can be trusted. It's important that you have a reliable compounding pharmacy with knowledgeable pharmacists if you decide to go this route.

Progesterone

If you have a uterus and are taking estrogen, you must take progesterone in some form or fashion to protect your uterine lining from growing wild and out of control and turning into uterine cancer. The old standby for this purpose is Provera. It is a powerful, synthetic progestagin that works well on the uterine lining. But I never prescribe this drug because it has three lousy and dangerous side effects. For example, it can increase your cholesterol, raise your blood pressure, and cause spasm of your blood vessels. As I mentioned earlier, a lot of doctors thought these are the reasons for more heart attacks and strokes in the women taking Prempro in the Women's Health Initiative.

When I prescribe progesterone, it's usually in the form of Prometrium. Prometrium is a natural micronized progesterone pill derived from wild yams and set in a peanut oil base. (If you're allergic to peanuts, you shouldn't take this drug.) It is made by a large pharmaceutical company and prescribed by a doctor. It's often covered by health insurance plans. It can make women sleepy, but if taken before bed, they may appreciate that side effect.

For some women, progesterone either in the form of Provera or Prometrium can make them feel fatigued or bloated, or cause headaches and even depression. Those women may do well to take vaginal progesterone, such as Prochieve vaginal gel 4 percent. Again, this is bio-identical progesterone like Prometrium, but it is placed in the vagina every other night for twelve nights (six doses) every month, every other month, or every third month, depending on her HRT program. By being absorbed in the vaginal mucosa (skin of the vagina), the liver can be bypassed and many side effects can be avoided. It's a little messier than a pill, of course, but for some women the trade-off is worth it.

Will I Have a Period If I Take Hormones?

When you take hormones after menopause, you will continue to menstruate as you did before menopause. I'm always surprised by women's opinions of having periods. Some women want to because it makes them feel young or they feel they need to "clean out"; other women think of having a period as a curse and adamantly refuse to do it. If you've been in menopause for some time, you can usually choose to have a period once a month, once every other month, or once every third month. The period probably will be heavier the longer you wait in between, because the uterus has had that much more time to build up a thickened lining. Or you could choose to have no period at all by taking estrogen and progesterone together every day. Either way is fine with me; both have been found to be safe. It is simply a personal preference.

How Long Do I Stay on Hormones?

Like any drug, you always want the smallest effective dose for the shortest amount of time. Every year the dose and form of hormones should be reevaluated. One scenario I commonly see is when a woman comes in to me complaining of breast tenderness. She tells me she's been on the same dose of estrogen for the last ten years and can't understand why things have changed. Well, we all change with time. At twenty-two, our bucket of estrogen is huge and we are tremendously fertile. When we're thirty-two, we still have a large bucket, but at forty-two the bucket's beginning to shrink. When we're fifty-two it has shrunk a lot, and by sixty-two it barely holds a drop.

We become more sensitive to estrogen as we grow older. Less is more. The same dose that worked at fifty years old is overkill

THE GOOD, THE BAD, AND THE UGLY: Menopause – The Heat Goes On

for the same woman ten years later. The doses, along with forms of estrogen, should be reevaluated annually, and estrogen should be weaned down over time. Eventually, hot flashes subside and women may require only a small dose of vaginal estrogen for lubrication and nothing more. Safety is always my first concern with hormones; how long to stay on, which kinds, and what doses. Barring the issue of safety, however, how you want to handle your menopause—waiting it out, food and herbs, exercise, hormone replacement, or a combination approach—is up to you. At the end of the day, it's your body.

In some ways, I feel that my discussion about menopause is a little depressing and even a bit scary. But I don't want you to feel bad. All women go through menopause; it's a natural part of our lives. Some women fear it because it means they are getting older. But that's a good thing! You can't go backward, and you don't want to stop here. You can go forward armed with knowledge, healthy habits, and a good attitude. You weren't crazy about all parts of your childhood, adolescence, and childbearing years, were you? As you grow through the transition of menopause, you have wisdom that only age and experience can bring you. Use that wisdom to be healthy and happy in the second half of your life!

CHAPTER 10

BUST YOUR BUTT, NOT YOUR HIP:
Bone Up on Osteoporosis

Thoughts from Mary Jo:

As I have mentioned, I have osteopenia, which is just one step away from osteoporosis. Fortunately, I have kept my bone health stable, but not without some work.

It is imperative that persons with osteoporosis or osteopenia do weight-bearing movements. I won't say you don't have a choice, because you do. You can choose to do weight-bearing movements or you can choose not to. The choice not to will make your life miserable, but it is a choice.

Just recently I have begun wearing a weighted vest when I walk. My husband says I look like I'm going off to war because it looks very much like the body armor soldiers wear. I tell him I am going off to war—I am at war with bone loss and it is a war I intend to win. Dr. Sahni will explain how you can win that war.

What the Doctor Has to Say: Jyotsna Sahni, M.D.

Bone Up on Osteoporosis

There's nothing sadder than going to the mall and seeing a little white-haired old woman who is bent over in pain from osteoporosis of the spine. She's probably walking with a tripod cane—or worse, with a walker. She looks frail and vulnerable. As a preventive medicine doctor for women, nothing makes me madder. Osteoporosis is easily preventable; there's a simple, painless test to detect it early and lots of effective treatment available.

Osteoporosis (which simply means "porous bone") has become a national epidemic. It is an equal-opportunity disease, but it hits women harder than men. Of the ten million osteoporotic people in the United States, eight million are women! There are another thirty-four million people who have low bone mass and are at risk for osteoporosis. As our population ages, bone loss will become more and more prevalent. Its costs, in terms of both dollars and health, are steep. In 2002, the estimated national direct care expenditures for osteoporotic fractures, including hospitals, nursing homes, and outpatient services, was eighteen billion dollars!

One in two women over the age of fifty will have an osteoporotic fracture in her remaining lifetime. We have 206 bones in our bodies, but as we age, fractures of the spine and hips are probably the most important to avoid, with wrist and rib fractures close behind. If you break your little finger, I'm sorry, but it'll heal in four to six weeks. If you break your back, that's a disaster. Collapsed vertebrae can cause severe back pain and loss of height, and can lead to stooped posture. If you break your hip, that's a tragedy. A woman's risk of hip fracture is equal to her combined risk of breast, uterine, and ovarian cancer. In fact, women with a hip fracture are at a fourfold greater risk of a second one. At six months after a hip fracture, only 15 percent of patients can walk across a room unaided. Obviously, bone fractures don't just cost money, they cost us our independence and mobility.

Risk Factors for Bone Loss

There are numerous risk factors for bone loss. Some we can change, others we cannot. They include:

- Being female
- Being Caucasian or Asian
- Low bone density
- Personal history of fracture after the age of fifty
- Family history of fracture or osteoporosis
- Advanced age
- Thin or small frame
- Estrogen deficiency caused by menopause, especially early or surgically induced
- Loss of periods (amenorrhea)
- Hyperthyroidism
- Anorexia nervosa
- Low calcium intake (i.e., lactose intolerance)
- Deficiency of vitamin D
- Certain medications (i.e., steroids, methotrexate, anticonvulsants, antacids containing aluminum, cyclosporine, heparin, cholestyramine, gonadotropin releasing hormones, excess thyroid hormone, acid suppressing drugs, and SSRI antidepressant drugs, etc.)
- Sedentary lifestyle
- Cigarette smoking
- Excessive alcohol intake
- Excessive caffeine intake

Detection

Osteoporosis is often called a "silent" disease, meaning that there are no symptoms of the bone loss until you actually break a bone. You can't feel your bones getting thinner, so you don't know you have bone loss until it's too late. Fortunately, there are simple ways to measure bone density well before it gets out of control. Central testing measures the hip and the spine, while peripheral tests measure the finger, wrist, kneecap, shin, or heel bones. I use the DEXA scan (Dual X-ray Absorptiometry) on my patients. I scan the low back or lumbar spine and both hips with this minimal X-ray technique. It is absolutely painless and I get instant results.

I compare a woman's bone density to the average thirty-year-old woman in America. This comparison is known as the T-score. You might say, "Hey, I'm not thirty! That's not fair!" But it is fair: by thirty, you're as good as you're going to get. We lay down the most bone during mid-puberty. Those years are the most important in our lives for building density. If we're lucky, we'll hold on to our bones until we reach menopause.

At menopause, with the loss of estrogen, we will lose 1 to 4 percent of bone each year for about seven to ten years. These years will be our greatest loss and then the bone loss will slow down. If you are starting out with bone to spare, you will be fine. If you are starting out with marginal bone mass, you will likely end up with a fracture that could impair your quality of life. It's imperative to know your starting point so we will know how aggressive treatment needs to be. Medicare doesn't begin to pay for bone density tests for the average woman until she's sixty-five years old. By then, it may be too late. I recommend having a bone density test done at the age of forty, typically before any menopausal changes have occurred. This provides your doctor with a baseline bone density score so that a game plan can be formulated for your bone health.

In addition to the younger adult comparison, I also compare patients to a woman of the same age, race, and weight, a comparison known as your Z-score. But if you're ninety-nine years old, I don't really care how you compare to your bingo partners; by then all women have lost a lot of bone. I want to know how you compare against the best bones, those of young women. The World Health Organization defines osteopenia as one standard deviation below the average young adult woman, or a T-score of -1.0 to -2.4. You can think of -1.0 as 90 percent of the bone density of a thirty-year-old.

BUST YOUR BUTT, NOT YOUR HIP: Bone Up on Osteoporosis

The WHO defines osteoporosis as -2.5 or worse. A T-score of -2.5 is having only 75 percent of the bone of an average thirty-year-old woman. These definitions help doctors decide when drugs, in addition to supplements, may be necessary to treat bone loss.

Calcium

Calcium is the main bone mineral and we need to get enough, either from food or supplements, to provide us the building blocks for bone. Of all the calcium in the body, 99 percent is in our bones and teeth. Calcium also plays a role in the function of muscles, the heart, hormones, and the nervous system. First, how much do we need? Table 1 (calcium requirements for age) addresses this.

Where do we get calcium? We can get it from food. Many foods contain calcium, especially dairy foods. See table 2 (calcium in foods). It is important to note that calcium absorption decreases with age, and also from a high-fiber diet and low levels of estrogen, vitamin D, or stomach acid. A diet that produces high acidity in the blood, such as a high-protein, Atkins-type diet, can cause calcium to leach from your bones.

When you can't get enough calcium from food, you may have to rely on calcium in supplements. There are basically two kinds: calcium carbonate and calcium citrate.

Calcium carbonate is cheap, easy, and available. Common name brands include Oscal, Caltrate, or Tums. However, it requires stomach acid to absorb well. If you are over the age of sixty, you are likely to make less stomach acid than a younger person, so calcium carbonate would not be recommended for you. If you take acid-suppressing drugs, such as H2 blockers like Pepcid or proton pump inhibitions such as Prilosec, you should not take calcium carbonate. If you have a delicate stomach and suffer from gas, bloating, or constipation, calcium carbonate may exacerbate your symptoms. If you have significant bone loss, calcium carbonate may simply be less well absorbed, so again it may not be your best bet. If you are clear to take calcium carbonate, take it with food, as that's when the stomach acids are doing their thing, helping to digest your food and absorb your calcium.

For all calcium supplements, do not take more than 500 mg at one sitting. Your gut simply can't absorb more. Last week, a woman came into my office for her bone density test. She was feeling very smug; she told me not to worry because she took 1,200 mg of calcium a day—every morning first thing she swallowed six calcium pills! Ugh! Not only is this an unappetizing breakfast, but it was a waste of time, money, and effort. You can't absorb more than about 500 mg of calcium at one time, so you must divide your calcium doses throughout the day.

The other main form of calcium supplement is calcium citrate. This is a slightly larger molecule and a little more expensive. It's better for you if you are over age sixty, take an acid-blocking drug, have a delicate stomach, or have significant bone loss. You can take it with or without food because its absorption is less dependent on an acidic environment in the gut. You still should limit doses to no more than 500 mg at once. A common name brand is Citrical.

Calcium can cause gas, bloating, and constipation in some people. It's best to make sure you get enough water, fiber, and exercise when you take it. Also, you should gradually increase your dose. If you can, get calcium from food. It will be easier to digest. Keep a three-day food diary to see how much calcium you get from diet itself. If it's not enough, then start to supplement. Both calcium carbonate and calcium citrate come in pill, chewable, and liquid forms. The latter two are probably more easily absorbed.

Calcium can interfere with absorption of medications such as thyroid hormone and tetracycline. It may interfere with the absorption of iron, unless iron is taken with vitamin C or is calcium citrate. If a medication is to be taken on an empty stomach, it should not be taken with calcium supplements.

Coral calcium became popular a few years ago and was touted as a miracle cure for all that ails you. I do not recommend coral calcium on two counts. First, there have been reports of heavy metal contamination with lead. Second, damage to the world's coral reefs as a result of profiteering from false claims concerns me. I do not recommend calcium from unrefined oyster shell, bone meal, or dolomite either, again because of concerns of lead and other heavy metal toxins.

How Much Do We Need?

How much is too much calcium? More than 2,500 mg/day of calcium may lead to problems such as high calcium levels in the blood (hypercalcemia), kidney stones, kidney failure, and milk-alkali syndrome, as well as interference of absorption of other minerals, including zinc, magnesium, and phosphorus.

Vitamin D

Vitamin D helps us absorb calcium. In fact, only 10 to 15 percent of calcium is absorbed without adequate amounts of vitamin D. But the vitamin D story is much more complex and interesting than that. The name "vitamin D" is probably a misnomer because it's much more a steroid hormone than a vitamin. Low levels of vitamin D have been associated with eighteen different cancers, including breast, colon, and prostate (the big three in the U.S.!), in addition to lupus, multiple sclerosis, ulcerative colitis, and other autoimmune diseases that typically occur much more in women than men. Low levels have also been linked to problems with muscle power, balance, hypertension, and even depression! Vitamin D deficiency is a big deal, beyond the bone issue.

Where do we get vitamin D? Well, we have evolved to get it from the sun. First, the sun hits your skin, makes a chemical reaction in your liver, goes on to your kidneys, and then gets transformed so it is biologically active. However, if you are wearing sunscreen or clothing or sitting in the shade, you may not get enough sunshine.

The time of day, the season, air pollution or even window glass can affect sunshine levels. Interestingly, the darker your skin, the more sunshine you need. Melanin in dark skin protects the skin from cancer but may impede the skin from making vitamin D. The older you are, the less efficient you are at making vitamin D from sunshine. If you live north of Atlanta or Los Angeles during the winter months, you couldn't get enough sunshine if you tried because the sun's rays hit the earth at such a low angle that vitamin D cannot be produced by it. (Not that anyone would spend twenty minutes three times a week wearing no clothes and no sunscreen while sitting in the sun in Boston, where it's dark by four p.m. in December!)

Only a few foods contain vitamin D, such as fatty fish, egg yolks, liver, and vitamin-fortified foods. If we simply can't get enough from food or sun, where can we get it? Well, to start, all multivitamins contain vitamin D. The question is: is the dose adequate for you? The best way to answer this question is with a simple blood test of vitamin D. This is especially true if you know you have any bone loss, because then you absolutely need to maximize your calcium absorption.

When I started reading about the vitamin D story in my medical journals, I immediately went out and tested myself (l love taking blood tests—I'm kind of an information junkie when it comes to my own health). That same month of September, I did bone density tests on five women who ended up with the diagnosis of osteopenia or osteoporosis. I told them that low bone mass was associated with low vitamin D. Could I check their vitamin D levels? They said yes. During the same month, I came across four patients who were breast cancer survivors and told them that breast cancer was associated with vitamin D. Could I check their levels? They too said yes. At the end of the month, I had ten levels—mine and my nine patients. I was fine (I have great bones, no family or personal history of cancer, and live in sunny Arizona); the other nine women were seriously low.

BUST YOUR BUTT, NOT YOUR HIP: Bone Up on Osteoporosis

I went to the grocery store, picked up vitamin D off the shelf and looked at the bottle: at one hundred tablets for four dollars, vitamin D is dirt cheap. But here's the caveat: unlike vitamin C, which is a water-soluble vitamin allowing excess to be spilled out in urine, vitamin D is fat-soluble and can literally poison you if you take too much. But how much is too much? It seems that less than 2,000 IU daily is probably safe for most of us. The National Osteoporosis Foundation recommends 400–800 IU daily. For some, this may be much too little. In the last couple of years, I have measured hundreds of vitamin D levels; most are too low. Again, testing your blood level is the best way to know what you need.

Other minerals and vitamins are also important in bone formation, but to a lesser extent. These include magnesium, zinc, boron, silica, and vitamin K, which can be obtained from both a well-balanced diet and supplements.

Exercise for Bone Health

Bones form our skeletons and hold up our bodies. They are made of minerals held together with collagen glue, with marrow in the middle. They are not overly sophisticated organs. We think of them as solid, but they are dynamic and change according to what we ask of them. Like muscles, which grow larger and stronger with weight training, bones grow stronger and denser when we ask them to work for us, too.

There are two main exercises for bones. The first is called weight-bearing. These are simply exercises where our bones hold up our weight, like walking, dancing, running, jumping rope, or step aerobics. Anywhere our bones and muscles have to fight gravity is weight-bearing. When we swim, the water holds us up; when we cycle, the bike holds us up. Neither swimming nor cycling is weight-bearing exercise; both provide good cardiovascular training and burn calories, but neither strengthens our bones.

The other exercise for bones is resistance training, such as weight lifting with free weights or on machines. Here, by resisting weight, we strengthen bone and increase muscle mass. If you have significant bone loss or are frail, you must be cautious with the exercises you choose. Certain movements like crunching or twisting the spine or high-impact aerobics could cause damage to delicate bones. Consult a knowledgeable health-care practitioner to guide you.

When I talk about exercise for bone health, I always include balance training. Why? Because when you are ninety I don't expect you to have the bone density of a thirty-year-old, but you need not fall when you get up at three a.m. to use the bathroom and trip over the dog in the dark. I can't tell you how many women I used to take care of like that back in my hospital days. Even back then I would get upset because I knew most of these injuries were preventable. Prevention is clearly the best medicine. Balance training includes dancing, yoga, and racket sports with quick hand-eye coordination. It also includes on-the-ball exercises, or simply standing on one foot in the morning when you brush your teeth and standing on the opposite foot at night when you brush your teeth again.

Sometimes you can incorporate balance training right into your weight workout. If you are doing bicep curls on one foot, it makes that fifteen-pound weight so much heavier if you must engage your core muscles to balance yourself. If I wanted to train for a marathon it might take many months, but to improve balance may take only three weeks. Balance is the easiest of the fitness parameters to improve in the shortest time; it's just as important as endurance and strength.

Fall Prevention

In addition to having good balance, we can improve our chances at fall prevention by making some simple changes. To avoid common hazards, take a look at this checklist.

BUST YOUR BUTT, NOT YOUR HIP: Bone Up on Osteoporosis

1) **Floors**

   Make sure throw rugs are secure. Remove loose wires, cords, and other clutter. Don't rearrange furniture too often.

2) **Bathrooms**

   Install grab bars in the shower and tub. Make sure the shower and tub have nonslip mats or tape. Make sure there are secure bath mats to dry wet, slippery feet.

3) **Lighting**

   Make sure areas both inside and outside the house are well-lit—driveways, walkways, front door, porches, hallways, bathrooms. Use night-lights in hallways to the bathroom and in the bathroom itself for nighttime safety.

4) **Kitchen**

   Mop up spills promptly. Install nonskid mats near the sink and stove.

5) **Shoes**

   Make sure shoes are stable. Dispense with unstable fashion (flimsy high heels or backless shoes and slippers) and replace with secure, comfortable shoes. This is even more important in the winter, when freezing rain and sleet can make sidewalks and roads more slippery and dangerous.

6) **Medications**

   Certain medications like sedatives, sleeping pills, muscle relaxants, and blood pressure drugs can contribute to dizziness and make you more unsteady on your feet. Speak to your doctor about these.

7) **Poor vision**

   Proper prescriptions for eyeglasses and adequate lighting help prevent falls.

8) **Poor hearing**

   Hearing aids can help you become more aware of your surroundings.

9) **Alcohol**

   Be conservative about alcohol use; don't overdo.

10) **Illness**

    Certain medical conditions such as Parkinson's disease or stroke can take a toll on our ability to balance and should be treated appropriately.

Medications for Bone Loss

While proper exercise, diet, and supplements are the best steps to take for bone loss prevention, medications can play a role where significant bone loss has already taken place.

Bones are made up of two main types of cells: osteoblasts and osteoclasts. The osteoblasts build bone while osteoclasts tear it down. There is constantly a building-up and breaking-down process going on in all our bones. When the breaking down is more prominent, we end up with a net loss of bone. Depending upon the severity of loss, we call this either osteopenia ("thinning bone") or osteoporosis ("porous bone"). While calcium must be present to provide building blocks for bone formation and vitamin D allows calcium to be absorbed by the body, sometimes adequate amounts of each simply don't keep up with the demands of the body and net bone loss occurs. Several drugs help stop the breakdown of bones so the building can occur effectively. These are called anti-resorptive agents.

The first is bisphosphonate therapy. These drugs act by slowing down osteoclastic activity, allowing osteoblasts to do their job, thereby increasing bone density. They also have been shown to decrease both vertebral and non-vertebral fractures and are used for prevention as well as treatment of osteoporosis. The most widely used examples of drugs in this category are Fosamax (alendronate) and Actonel (risendronate). These are often taken in a convenient once-weekly dosing schedule and are approved for both men and women. Fosamax seems to be effective for at least ten years.

Recently, Boniva (ibandronate) has joined the others, and is unique in that it may be taken only once monthly. These drugs are taken in pill form first thing in the morning on an empty stomach. They can cause reflux (irritation of the throat), so patients are warned to stay upright for one hour after swallowing the pill. While there have been recent concerns about these drugs causing osteonecrosis of the jaw (death of the cells of the jawbone) and poor healing after a fracture, bisphosphonates are generally tolerated well.

Another treatment is Miacalcin (salmon calcitonin). Administered as a nasal spray or by injection, this option has few side effects but unfortunately poor effectiveness. It may increase spinal density by directly inhibiting osteoclastic activity, but it has no significant effect at the hips. Interestingly, it may have an analgesic effect that makes it useful in the case of painful vertebral crush fractures.

Estrogen/progesterone also increase bone density and reduces fracture risk in postmenopausal women. The Women's Health Initiative showed a 33 percent reduction in vertebral fracture and 23 percent in others. Since hormone replacement therapy may be associated with increased incidence of breast cancer, strokes, blood clots, and possible heart attacks, it is not considered first line therapy in osteoporosis treatment.

Evista (raloxifene) is a selective estrogen receptor modulator (SERM) and may be used in postmenopausal bone loss. It does not work quite as well as estrogen, but it also increases bone density and reduces fracture risk. It is administered in a pill of 60 mg taken once a day. Interestingly, it appears to decrease the risk of estrogen-dependant breast cancer by 65 percent over four years. In addition, it may decrease total and LDL cholesterol values and does not cause vaginal bleeding and thickening of the uterine lining. Like estrogen, it works synergistically with bisphosphonates.

Forteo (recombinant human parathyroid hormone) is unique in that it actually stimulates bone growth rather than simply slowing bone breakdown. It helps the building cells of bone work better. It's the most powerful drug we've seen yet. Its efficacy exceeds what is seen in bisphosphonates and it works in both sexes. In post-menopausal women, fracture reduction has been seen in the spine, hip, foot, ribs, and wrist. Expensive and administered in daily injections for up to two years, Forteo should be reserved for high-risk patients only.

What Do You Need to Do to Help Your Bones?

- Eat a diet that is rich in calcium and vitamin D
- Do resistance training, weight-bearing exercise, and balance training regularly
- Live a healthy lifestyle—don't smoke or drink too much coffee or alcohol
- Stay up-to-date with regular bone density tests
- Remember, prevention is the best medicine!

Table 1: Calcium Needs By Age

Age group calcium needs in milligrams (mg.)

Infants
Birth to 6 months	210
6-12 months	270

Children/Young Adults
1-3 years	500
4-8 years	800
9-18 years	1,300

Adult Women and Men
19-50 years	1,000
50 + years	1,200

Pregnant or Lactating
18 years or younger	1,300
19-50 years	1,000

Source: National Academy of Sciences, 1997

Table 2: Calcium in Foods

Food Groups	Low Calcium Content (75 to 149 mg)	Moderate Calcium Content (150 to 249 mg)	High Calcium Content (> 250 mg)
Milk Group	· Cottage cheese, 2% 1/2 cup · Ice cream, ice milk	· Cheeses, 1 oz: · American processed · Brick · Caraway · Cheddar · Colby · Edam · Monterey Jack · Mozzarella, part skim · Meunster · Swiss processed	· Milks, 1 cup: · Buttermilk · Chocolate · Whole, 2%, 1% · Fortified Soy · Cheeses, 1 oz: · Ricotta, part skim · Swiss · Yogurt, low fat, 1 cup
Meat & Meat Substitutes	· Beans, cooked, 1 cup · Oysters, raw, 7 to 9 · Shrimp, raw, canned, 30 oz · Shrimp, fresh to 1 cup · Tofu, 4 oz. processed with calcium sulfate	· Salmon with bones, 3 oz	· Sardines with bones, 3 oz
Fruits & Vegetables	· Broccoli, 1 stalk · Dark leafy greens, 1/2 cup: · Bok choy, · spinach, · frozen collards, · kale, · okra, · mustard, · beet & turnip greens	· Collards, raw, 1/2 cup · Rhubarb, 1/2 cup	· Orange Juice, 1 cup fortified with calcium
Grains	· Cornbread (2.5 x 2.5 x 1.5 inch) · Corn tortillas (2) · Pancakes, 4" diameter (2) · Sesame seeds or Tahini, 1/4 cup	· Waffle, 7" diameter (1)	

CHAPTER 11

HOW TO STAY YOUNG AT HEART:
Women and Heart Disease

Thoughts from Mary Jo:

It came late one night—that phone call no one wants to get. "They've taken your father to the hospital," the voice on the other end of the line said. "He probably had a heart attack." By the time I got to the hospital, he was gone.

Heart disease kills 432,000 men in this country each year.[8] But what about women? We have all learned to be alert to breast cancer, but the scary little secret most women don't know is that the number-one killer of women is not breast cancer but heart disease. We are even better at it than men, I am not proud to say. Heart disease kills 499,000 women each year.[9]

But, hark! Like most of the women's health issues that we discuss in this book, there is much we, as women, can do to reverse this trend. Next, Dr. Sahni is going to "get to the heart of the matter."

What the Doctor Has to Say: Jyotsna Sahni, M.D.

Most Americans know that heart disease is the number-one killer of men in the United States. What most Americans don't know is that heart disease is also the number-one killer of women over the age of twenty-five in the United States[10]—more than breast cancer. In fact, heart disease kills more women than breast cancer, uterine cancer, and ovarian cancers combined. About five hundred thousand women die each year of clogged arteries. This translates to one death each minute. But death is NOT the only thing that should concern you. Today, medical technology and medicines are very effective at keeping you alive despite heart disease, but the quality of your life can become greatly reduced. For every person who dies of heart disease, many more are living for years in a poor state of health. How do you want to spend your "golden" years?

Women are different from men in so many ways; why would we manifest heart disease in the same way? We all probably know that crushing chest pain or having an "elephant" sitting on the chest is a sign of a heart attack. When that occurs, it's obvious that something bad is happening and an urgent call to 911 is required. What women don't often realize is that the "classic" symptoms that warn of a heart attack in a woman may be different than the description we've been given of a heart attack that occurs in men: crushing pain, tingling down the left arm or up the jaw, or shortness of breath.

Women can have a heart attack like this too, but they may also simply feel fatigued, dizzy, sweaty, or nauseated. Since the symptoms may be more subtle, women tend to delay getting medical attention. By the time a woman gets to the emergency room, it may be too late. Many women disregard the seriousness of feeling bad and miss a critical opportunity to be helped. In the past, doctors were just as likely as women themselves to push off vague symptoms as stress, but today most doctors are tuned-in to the differences between men and women. Unfortunately, the word just hasn't gotten out to most women. Just as in the case of breast cancer, early detection of a heart attack can lead to better survival.

Women differ from men not just in the symptoms of their heart attacks but also in when they occur. Most women develop heart disease about ten years later than men. Since they may be frailer or suffer from multiple medical problems at an older age, they tend to do worse with heart disease than men. For example, more women than men will die the first year after having a heart attack. Black women are at an even greater disadvantage, and are less likely than men or white women to receive life-saving therapies for heart attacks. Prevention is important. Two-thirds of women who have a heart attack fail to make a full recovery.

If a woman is in menopause, it affects her risk of heart disease. Of course, menopause tracks with age, but estrogen poses a distinct advantage to women when it comes to heart disease. I could take two women who are both fifty-five years old, one of whom went into menopause at the age of fifty and the other who is still getting regular periods. The one who had an earlier menopause may have higher blood pressure, worse cholesterol (the "lousy" LDL goes up and the "healthy" HDL goes down), less elasticity of blood vessels, and increased clotting risk. In short, the menopausal woman is at higher risk for heart disease even though both women are the same chronological age. It seems that hormone replacement would provide an easy antidote, but unfortunately the effects of hormones are complex and the decision to use them must be well thought out and individualized for a woman's overall health. (Please refer to chapter 9 – The Good, the Bad, and the Ugly: Menopause.)

What Is a Heart Attack?

Your heart is merely a muscular pump the size of your fist that delivers blood to all your body organs. When the blood vessels that feed oxygen and nutrients to your heart fail, then your heart muscle cries out in pain (or fatigue, nausea, dizziness, etc.). If an area of heart muscle isn't fed for long enough, it dies. That's a heart attack. If it's a little piece of heart muscle, you'll survive it. If it's the main pumping chamber of the heart that's hit, then it could kill.

What Causes Heart Disease?

There are numerous risk factors for heart disease. It damages the blood vessels to the heart, encouraging cholesterol plaque to adhere to the vessel walls. Doctors used to think of a heart attack like clogged pipes in the kitchen sink. They assumed that there had to be a lot of cholesterol buildup before blood vessels were clogged and a heart attack would happen. Now we know that clogged arteries are important, but even a small amount of cholesterol plaque, even a 20 to 30 percent blockage, can be deadly when combined with inflammation. Inflammation irritates the small piece of cholesterol plaque on the inside of the blood vessel wall and causes it to rupture. The body interprets the ruptured plaque like an injury and makes a clot that then cuts off blood circulation to the heart muscle.

What Are Risk Factors for Heart Disease?

Age

The older we are, the more likely we are to get heart disease. This is one of those risk factors you can't change. You don't want to stop here, and you can't go backward. Aging is inevitable, but healthy aging is up to you.

Family History

Heart disease tends to run in families. While you can't change your parents (no matter how much you might like to), you can change how you treat your body.

Smoking

Smoking ages the blood vessels prematurely. Smokers' blood vessels are older than those of people the same age who don't smoke. Smoking increases your risks for many cancers, hurts the lungs, makes you look old, and increases inflammation and blood pressure. Even secondhand smoke is dangerous. Smoking while taking the birth control pill is especially problematic because it makes you even more likely to have a stroke, heart attack, and high blood pressure. Please don't smoke.

Diabetes

Diabetes is a disease that is defined by high blood sugar. In fact, the medical definition of diabetes is two fasting blood sugars on different days above 125 mg/dl. There are two types of diabetes. The first is type 1, which used to be called "juvenile" diabetes because it typically appeared in childhood. This is the disease in which the pancreas fails and stops making insulin, the hormone that packages away blood sugar into the body's cells. Type 1 requires four or five shots of insulin each day. It does increase the risk for heart disease but is not a risk factor we can avoid.

Type 2 diabetes, also referred to as "adult onset" diabetes or "old age" diabetes, has become a rising epidemic in the United States as the population has grown older and fatter. The actual diagnosis of diabetes is preceded by "insulin resistance," which is also termed "pre-diabetes," "metabolic syndrome," "dysmetabolic syndrome," "dysglycemia," or "glucose intolerance." In this process, the body becomes resistant to the effects of the hormone insulin, which is produced by the pancreas. As a result of the body's resistance to insulin, the pancreas must generate increasing amounts of insulin to overcome this resistance. Type 2 diabetes is often preventable (or at least manageable).

This is the kind of diabetes that tends to run in families and typically occurs at older ages. First, you inherit the gene. You grow up. You gain weight, especially around your middle. This is known as "apple-shaped" obesity. While chubby thighs and a big butt are no fun, they are mostly a cosmetic concern. Fat around the belly and around the body organs is downright dangerous. This "visceral" fat is more associated with diabetes, heart disease, stroke, and even cancer. Many women notice a "middle-age spread" around menopause. They look less like an hourglass shape and more like a rectangle, having lost their tiny waists. It's not always easy to lose weight or even maintain one's weight, but for women with a predisposition toward diabetes, doing so can be life-saving.

As the diabetic process unfolds, cholesterol values change in predictable ways. Triglycerides, the least important part of cholesterol, begin to rise. HDL (the "healthy" cholesterol) falls. Blood pressure begins to climb and blood sugars go up. It's at this point that most doctors diagnose diabetes. But diabetes is a slow, predictable process and if we catch it early we can stop it early. Women with diabetes increase their risk for heart disease by **three times!**

Preventing and controlling diabetes with lifestyle changes is amazingly effective. First, avoid sugar. It doesn't take a rocket scientist to understand that if diabetes is a disease of too much sugar, we should eat less of it. Sugar is EVERYWHERE: honey, maple syrup, cake, candy, cola, bread, rice, pasta, and alcohol. (Yes, alcohol is the same as sugar to the body, sorry.) Less is more. When you choose to indulge in that sweet treat, make sure you combine it with a fat, protein, and fiber to blunt the effect of the sugar. For example, if it's four o'clock on a Saturday afternoon and you get hungry, open the refrigerator, and spy a piece of chocolate cake calling out your name—I beg you, don't do it! If there's nothing else in your belly, the sugar from that cake will make your blood sugar spike, along with your insulin levels. An hour or two later you may feel shaky, sick, tired, moody, and literally fatter (because high insulin levels signal the body to lay down fat).

On the other hand, if you have the same chocolate cake after a dinner of salmon and broccoli, it will have a much different metabolic effect. The salmon is a good source of protein and healthy omega-3 fats (ocean salmon is far healthier than farm-raised "Atlantic salmon"); the broccoli provides you with water, fiber, and cancer-fighting nutrients. Now the very same chocolate cake hurts you less. If you know you'll be having cake for dessert, plan to skip the bread or pasta. No one, especially if you are diabetic or pre-diabetic, needs a bunch of "high" glycemic index carbohydrates. Fruits and vegetables, yes; refined or processed carbs, no.

Second, to avoid diabetes, exercise. Every time you exercise, you burn sugar. The sugar-burning effect of exercise lasts twenty-four to thirty hours. How often should you exercise if you are diabetic or want to avoid diabetes? (Lu Jurcova Phillips discusses exercise in chapter 4.) But my philosophy, based on that math, is very simple: exercise most days of the week. If all you've got is ten minutes of time, energy, or interest, exercise for ten minutes and give your body a soft message of "burn sugar." If you're out on a sunny Saturday morning with your best friend and want to hike hard for two hours, give your body a loud message of "BURN SUGAR!" Like the Nike ads say, "*Just Do It!*"

Third, lose weight. For most people, weight loss really helps prevent and even treat diabetes. As I said earlier, it may be lifesaving.

High Blood Pressure

High blood pressure, or "hypertension," is just what it sounds like—high pressure in the blood vessels of the body. The small blood vessels are most vulnerable, like the ones in your head. High blood pressure is a major risk factor for stroke. Strokes are the number-one cause of disability for Americans; if you can't get around, you lose your independence. No one wants a stroke. Damage to the small blood vessels in your eyes can lead to loss of vision. The blood vessels of your heart can be damaged by high pressures, leading to heart failure and heart attack. Uncontrolled blood pressure is a major cause of kidney failure. In men, high blood pressure damages small vessels in the penis, leading to impotence.

For years, hypertension was called the "silent" killer. This is because we can't feel our blood pressures (most of the time). You simply have to measure it. Blood pressure has two numbers. The top number is the systolic and measures the squeeze of the heart as it sends clean blood to all the body organs. The bottom is the diastolic that represents the pause of the heart when it fills with clean blood before it pumps again. Both numbers are important. An ideal pressure is 120/80 (or less) at rest. When you exercise hard, are fighting with your teenager, or get cut off in traffic, the body is stressed and your blood pressure may go up temporarily. That's okay, as long as it doesn't go too high for too long.

There are some natural ways to drop blood pressure. First, if you smoke, quit. Among other bad things, smoking raises blood pressure. Next, quit drinking too much alcohol. Eating less salt can help those who are salt sensitive. Wherever salt goes, water follows. If you ate a bag of potato chips last night, you may find your rings and shoes are too tight today and your weight is up a few pounds. You've held on to extra fluid. Extra fluid in your blood vessels translates to higher blood pressure. Stress makes you pump out adrenaline, which also can raise blood pressure.

Stress reduction practices such as meditation, yoga stretching, and yogic breathing may help lower blood pressure. Extra weight may make blood pressure rise; weight loss can help. Regular exercise also can help lower blood pressure. Although blood pressure rises at the time of a workout, with conditioning, the body's blood vessels get better at dilating or opening up, and eventually blood pressure improves. If lifestyle measures fail at getting your blood pressure down to a good number, fortunately there are many great drugs that can help. Blood pressure needs to be measured regularly and controlled well.

High Cholesterol

Cholesterol is made in the liver. The degree to which the cholesterol in your body becomes a risk factor for heart disease depends on both your genetics and your lifestyle. There are skinny marathon runners who eat nothing but twigs and grass and have high cholesterol because they have lousy genes and over-productive livers. Most of us, however, will improve our cholesterol numbers with better diets, weight control, and exercise.

Cholesterol is an important risk factor for heart disease, but only one among many. It has gotten a lot of press in the last few years, probably much more than it deserves, only because drug companies have a drug to control it. Many doctors follow the National Cholesterol Education Program guidelines for cholesterol last put forth by the National Heart, Lung, and Blood Institute in 2004. They say that you should have a total cholesterol value under 200 mg/dl. I say the total number is really not as important as the breakdown of the whole. The component parts of cholesterol are what matter more. For example, the LDL (or "lousy") cholesterol should be as low as possible. Excess LDL clogs up arteries. Keeping saturated and trans fats to a minimum in your diet can lower LDL, as can a diet high in fiber. If you have zero or one heart risk factors, your LDL should be under 160 mg/dl. If you have two or more risk factors, your LDL should be under 130 mg/dl. If you have heart disease (or if you have had a heart attack, stent, angioplasty, bypass, etc.), you should be under 100 mg/dl.

Because cholesterol medicines are so effective at lowering cholesterol, doctors have become much more aggressive at using these to lower LDL. As a result, there have been more and more *side effects* of cholesterol medications reported: muscle and joint aches, depression, dry skin/eczema, memory problems, liver irritation. No drug is perfectly safe. If you are at high risk for heart disease, drugs may be the best prescription if nothing else has worked. Too often the drugs become the first approach. Cardiologists have told me that they rarely see patients willing to adopt the lifestyle changes necessary to reduce their risk factors in a natural way; hence, the overuse of the drugs.

The other important cholesterol particle is the HDL or "healthy" cholesterol. The higher it is, the better it is. It should be at least 50 mg/dl. Exercise, weight loss (if necessary) and possibly adding nuts, soy, or olive oil to the diet may increase HDL. Sometimes niacin (vitamin B_3) is prescribed in huge doses and used as a drug to increase HDL.

Triglycerides may go up with high blood sugars, too much alcohol, extra weight, or oral estrogens like birth control pills or oral hormone replacement therapy. Triglycerides should be under 150 mg/dl. In addition to treating these predisposing factors to high triglycerides, large doses of fish oil may be prescribed to lower this part of cholesterol. After several months of healthy lifestyle changes, recheck cholesterol levels to look for improvements. Worst case scenario: your doctor may need to prescribe a drug for high cholesterol. But try all the healthy lifestyle changes first.

Inflammation

The high-sensitivity C-reactive protein and fibrinogen are markers of inflammation in the body. Inflammation is a key component of cardiac risk. Inflammation encourages cholesterol plaque that has developed upon the lining of a blood vessel to become unstable and rupture, thereby inciting a cascade of biochemical events that cause a heart attack. Without inflammation, cholesterol plaque poses less of a risk. Inflammation in the body can be partly ameliorated by the ingestion of omega-3 fatty acids, vitamins, anti-inflammatory herbs like ginger, turmeric, and mint, and foods such as berries, pumpkin seeds, and dark leafy greens. Reducing stress also can reduce inflammation.

Homocysteine

Homocysteine is a sticky protein in the blood that may damage blood vessel walls and encourage cholesterol plaque to lay down. It has been implicated in heart disease, stroke, cancer, osteoporosis, and Alzheimer's disease. It is easily reduced by the adequate intake of vitamins B_6, B_{12}, and folic acid.

Stress

Stress affects the balance between the sympathetic nervous system (the accelerator of the heart that makes it beat fast) and the parasympathetic nervous system (the brake pedal of the heart that slows it down). In a car, we want our accelerator and brake pedals to cooperate so we can negotiate traffic on the freeway. As a result, cars drive fast and slow as needed. In our hearts, we want the sympathetic and parasympathetic nervous systems to cooperate so we can negotiate stress in our lives. Obviously, if you are exercising, your heart rate goes fast. Deep in sleep at night, our heart rates slow down. But even if you are just sitting and reading this book, your heart rate will go up and down. Your heart rate varies. This is a good thing; the more it varies, the healthier it is for your heart. If we had our foot on just the gas, we would crash and burn. If we had our foot only on the brake pedal, we wouldn't get anywhere. With enough stress over enough time, our heart rate variability decreases and makes us vulnerable to an abnormal heart rhythm.

Stress makes other risk factors for heart disease worse. For example, if you are under stress, your blood pressure may go up, you may overeat and choose unhealthy foods, you may skip your exercise and be more likely to pick up a pack of cigarettes. Chronic stress exposes your body to stress hormones like adrenaline and cortisol which take a toll. When you are under stress, your platelets get stickier and your C-reactive protein and fibrinogen levels rise, making you more likely to develop a clot and therefore have a heart attack. It's critically important to find a way to reduce your stress. Exercise, good friends, laughter and having fun, thinking about life in an adaptive way, meditation, and breathing exercises can help.

Depression

Women suffer from depression more commonly than men. Symptoms include: feeling sad, hopeless, helpless, guilty, worthless, or restless; sleep disturbances; pain; fatigue; gaining or losing weight; and not finding pleasure in things that previously gave pleasure. Women with depression are more likely to have heart disease, and women who have heart disease and depression do worse with both. One in six patients who have had a heart attack suffers from depression. During recovery from heart surgery, depression can intensify pain, worsen fatigue, and decrease survival. Having depression also gets in the way of taking good care of yourself and your heart risk factors.

When people are depressed, they tend to isolate themselves from others, even people who love them. Family, friends, a supportive therapist, even a loving dog or cat is good for the heart—on so many levels. Depression can be successfully treated with exercise, nutritional supplements, sunshine, mind-body practices, therapy, and medication.

Poor Sleep

In recent years, studies have shown that sleep is critical to good health. Poor sleep is associated with higher blood pressure, higher blood sugar, extra weight, and obstructive sleep apnea—all risks factors for heart disease. Please see chapter 13 for a full discussion of sleep.

Sedentary Lifestyle/Obesity

Not exercising and extra weight significantly increase a woman's risk for heart disease. The good news is that it's never too late. You don't have to be a size 2; even a 5 to 10 percent weight loss will make a significant difference in blood pressure, blood sugar, and overall heart risk. Being fit even if you're carrying extra weight goes a long way toward protecting your heart.

Prevent Heart Disease

- Eat a diet with lots of colorful fruits and vegetables. Avoid saturated fats and trans fats, high sugar, and highly processed foods. Get enough fiber.

- Exercise regularly.
- Keep your body at a good weight.
- Get eight hours of sleep each night.
- Don't smoke.
- Practice a stress-reduction program, like meditation, yoga, and yogic breathing. Simple breathing practices can be done by anyone and recent studies are documenting significant benefits.
- Enjoy the company of friends, family, and a loving pet.
- See your doctor regularly to check blood pressure and for blood tests.

CHAPTER 12

EVERY WOMAN'S WORST FEAR:
The Ticking Time Bomb – Breast Cancer

Thoughts from Mary Jo:

I thankfully have never had breast cancer, but I have had the privilege to be a life coach for someone who did. "Diane" was an inspiration to me and those around her. I was her life coach, but she taught me more about life than I ever could have imagined.

Dr. McIntyre will set out the things you need to know about breast cancer, give you stories of women who have survived it, and offer some ways to reduce your risk of getting breast cancer.

My story to you from coaching Diane is that women have the capacity to be incredibly strong and to persevere. For her, it was several things: 1) she had a great doctor; 2) she kept a positive attitude; 3) she maintained her spiritual life; 4) she continued to exercise; and 5) she began eating mostly fruits and vegetables.

I am thrilled to report that she is very much alive ten years later.

What the Doctor Has to Say: Kristi McIntyre, M.D.

I am here to be the skunk at the garden party.

My co-authors have been telling you how important it is to eat right, exercise, lift weights, and stay positive. And they're right. All of these things are absolutely crucial to your long-term well-being and I second their recommendations wholeheartedly.

However, as a breast cancer specialist, I can tell you that I see women every day who did all the right things and still drew the short straw. They got cancer.

The truth is, many factors outside your control—such as age, gender, genetics, and environment—can determine your cancer risk. The good news, however, is that regardless of your breast cancer risk factors, early detection through various screening methods is almost entirely in your control. And that can literally mean the difference between life and death.

Let's talk about the "controllables" first, because there is little doubt that lifestyle choices play at least some role—in some cases, a significant role—in your breast cancer risk.

Diet

For decades, scientists have believed that lifestyle and nutrition influenced a woman's chance of developing breast cancer. The belief in part was due to clues obtained from observational studies comparing country-to-country differences in breast cancer rates.

Japanese women were observed to have significantly lower rates of breast cancer compared to similar women in America. Even more compelling was the observation that when Japanese women immigrated to the United States, after only two generations their breast cancer rates were the same as any other ethnic group. Naturally, the assumption was that something carcinogenic in the American diet or lifestyle must be the culprit contributing to the increased rates of breast cancer.

Obesity, possibly from increased dietary fat, was already established as elevating a woman's serum estrogen level. Prolonged estrogen exposure was known to increase breast cancer risk. Couple this with the fact that in the 1990s dietary fat was *the* nutritional evil of the decade, and it's easy to understand why fat became a focus of breast cancer prevention and research. Several studies were initiated to assess the impact of dietary fat and breast cancer.

The National Institutes of Health launched a series of clinical studies to address important questions regarding women's health. One such study was the Women's Health Initiative (WHI) Dietary Modification Trial. This was a large, ambitious trial with more than forty-eight thousand participants, designed to evaluate the effects of low dietary fat on breast cancer risk. The women included were all postmenopausal and randomly assigned to either a dietary change group or a comparison group, which maintained their usual eating habits.

The dietary modification participants met with nutritionists and attempted to reduce their total dietary fat to 20 percent of calories. The women were followed for eight years. At the conclusion, the women in the dietary change group had a 9 percent lower risk of breast cancer. This was considered only "marginally significant" and thus did not put to rest the connection between dietary fat and breast cancer.

As one can imagine, dietary studies are hard to conduct and implement. In the WHI study, although the women were supposed to limit their fat intake to 20 percent, they could only manage to limit it to 24 percent—which is still lower than most average Americans can manage. So, even if the study proved conclusively that extremely low levels of fat intake could reduce breast cancer risk, given the difficulty of maintaining such a diet, for all practical purposes it would do little to help average women reduce their risk.

Another study, the Women's Intervention Nutrition Study (WINS), was launched in 1992 with a different population of women who were highly motivated. These women all had developed breast cancer and had been treated with surgery, radiation, and chemotherapy. The goal of the study was to address whether a low-fat diet would lower the risk of breast cancer *recurrence.*

As with the WHI study, the women were either assigned to a fat reduction diet, with intensive one-on-one counseling with a nutritionist, or followed a standard diet. After eight years, the reduced fat group saw a 9.8 percent recurrence rate, and the standard diet group saw a 12.4 percent recurrence rate—a modest reduction, at best.

Another large, ambitious trial supporting the WHI and WINS trial is the National Institutes of Health-AARP Diet and Health Study, which started in 1987. In this study, 188,000 healthy, postmenopausal women filled out detailed surveys about their dietary habits. It was determined that women who consumed the lowest amount of fat had a 15 percent lower risk of developing breast cancer.

What, therefore, is the verdict on dietary fat as it pertains to breast cancer risk? Reducing dietary fat is a good idea for a number of health reasons—maintaining a healthy weight or reducing your risk of heart disease or stroke, for example—but I and my colleagues in the breast cancer field do not consider it a surefire way to ensure you do not become one of our patients.

Obesity

While there is a link between the fat you put *in* you and breast cancer, there is substantially more evidence that the fat you carry *on* you can play a role in your breast cancer risk. Obesity has been associated with both an increased risk of developing breast cancer and a worse prognosis after onset of the disease.

Possible reasons for this link are still being studied, but some researchers speculate that it could be related to higher and longer lifetime exposure to estrogens in overweight individuals or elevation of insulin levels, which may stimulate the growth of breast cancer cells.

Because the link between obesity and increased breast cancer risk has been fairly well-established, I and my colleagues heartily recommend maintaining a healthy weight as an important step in lowering your risk for breast cancer and for improving your odds of survival if you have already developed it.

Aim for a BMI (body mass index) between 18.5 and 24.9. (See the chart at the back of this book to calculate your current and ideal BMI.)

Exercise

Oncologists are always looking for new strategies to prevent or treat breast cancer. Unfortunately, most of these strategies come at a price, both financially and in terms of lower quality of life. But one strategy seems to offer a win-win solution: exercise.

In one study, the Iowa Women's Health Study by the Mayo Clinic, researchers found that women who took part in vigorous activity two times a week (jogging, swimming, aerobics, etc.), or moderate activity four times a week (long walks, golfing, etc.) saw a 14 percent reduction in risk of developing breast cancer compared to those in the study who had a low level of physical activity.

Even more exciting is a study from Harvard Medical School that indicates women can boost their odds of beating breast cancer with moderate exercise. They analyzed nearly three thousand women who were treated with surgery, radiation, or chemotherapy for breast cancer. The women were asked how much they exercised and at what intensity. After ten years, 92 percent of women who exercised three to five hours a week (or thirty minutes a day) were still alive, compared to 86 percent who got less than one hour a week of physical exertion.

This means you don't have to run a marathon to improve your chances of beating (or preventing the onset of) breast cancer. Even moderate exercise helps, and it's free!

Alcohol

Alcohol consumption has consistently been linked to an increased risk of developing breast cancer. The American Cancer Society's Cancer Prevention Study reported that even one drink per day, on average, increased a postmenopausal woman's chance of dying from breast cancer by 30 percent, compared to women who did not consume alcohol.

Surprisingly, even modest amounts of alcohol seem to affect breast cancer risk. For the average woman who consumes one alcoholic drink a day, her chance of being diagnosed with breast cancer during her lifetime goes from one in eight to almost one in seven.

Countries with high alcohol consumption, such as Italy, have a higher incidence of breast cancer than countries with lower consumption rates. The type of alcohol—beer, wine, or liquor—seems to make no difference.

Of course, the correlation between alcohol consumption and breast cancer must be balanced with the recorded benefits of moderate alcohol consumption in preventing heart disease. All things considered, the occasional alcoholic beverage is unlikely to make a large difference in your breast cancer risk and it does pose benefits to your heart.

Soy

Can soy supplements or eating a soy-rich diet protect you from developing breast cancer? Maybe yes, maybe no. Interest in soy was energized by data suggesting that countries, such as Japan, whose populations eat a soy-rich diet, have fewer breast cancer cases.

However, caution must be used in interpreting this information as it relates to soy, since the traditional Japanese diet differs in many other ways from the Western diet. The traditional Japanese diet is also less processed and contains a wide variety and large quantity of fruits and vegetables, very little red meat, ample amounts of fish, and much smaller amounts of sweets—any one of which may play a role in the lower incidence of breast cancer in Japan. Additionally, the rate of obesity in Japan is much lower than in America—in large part because of their dietary habits, which also may help explain their lower breast cancer rates.

Indeed, research into whether soy is helpful or harmful has been conflicting. The existing research raises more questions than it answers. An analysis of eighteen different studies did not yield a statistically significant benefit to adding soy or soy supplements to your diet. And some animal studies have shown that soy can produce both a protective *and* a stimulatory effect on breast cancer cells.

The National Cancer Institute has an ongoing study on the effect of soy supplements on breast mammographic density, which seems to correlate with a higher risk of breast cancers.

Why the confusion? It could be the conflicting nature of soy itself. Soy is considered a "phytoestrogen," a group of substances derived from plants that are structurally and functionally similar to estrogen, high levels of which are linked to increased risk of breast cancer. However, studies in the 1980s showed a component of soy called "isoflavones" may actually *block* the body's own estrogens.

One of the reasons women are interested in soy is anecdotal evidence that it can help control menopausal symptoms, such as hot flashes. However, in clinical studies, soy supplements have not been shown to be any more effective than a placebo in reducing hot flashes.

The bottom line is there are currently no clear advantages or disadvantages, from a breast cancer perspective, to eating soy. More study is needed before a definitive answer can be given.

Nevertheless, it is probably safe to eat soy-based foods, such as tofu. Highly refined soy supplements, however, should probably be avoided.

Vitamin D

My personal favorite news story of late was titled "Sunshine Vitamin Wards Off Breast Cancer." It was my favorite because it was *true*, easy to implement, and had the real possibility of improving the health of American women. Two studies presented at the American Association of Cancer Research showed that women who consumed adequate amounts of vitamin D are less likely to develop breast cancer. In the first study, higher levels of vitamin D translated into a 50 percent reduction in breast cancer risk. The second study provided evidence that sun exposure between the ages of ten and nineteen, when breasts are developing, leads to a significant decrease in breast cancer risk.

Even more encouraging was a Canadian observational study that measured vitamin D levels in breast cancer survivors. Those with low levels were much more likely to recur and die of breast cancer.

Additionally, in the United States, it has long been observed that women who grow up in northern states have a higher incidence of breast cancer than those who live in "sunshine states" like Florida.

Vitamin D is contained in milk, salmon, tuna, and other oily fish. But we are unable to consume a sufficient amount from diet alone of the best type of vitamin D, which is vitamin D_3. Our bodies make vitamin D from sunlight, but sun exposure is controversial because of the skin cancer risk. Nevertheless, most people can safely get the ten to fifteen minutes of unprotected sun exposure a day without significantly increasing their risk of skin cancer. That ten- to fifteen-minute figure, incidentally, is for Caucasian women. African-Americans would need longer exposure to get a sufficient amount of vitamin D.

Health professionals are becoming more aware of the importance of vitamin D and are therefore monitoring it more frequently. In some cases, supplemental vitamin D may be recommended. If you're considering supplementing with vitamin D, shoot for 800 IU a day. And stay tuned as we learn more about the cancer-protective benefits of vitamin D.

Hormone Replacement Therapy

"Breast Cancer Rates Decline Sharply," declared a headline reporting the NCI's analysis of data from the Surveillance, Epidemiology, and End Results (SEER) registries. That analysis showed that the rate of breast cancer in American women fell sharply in 2003 as compared to 2002. The decline began in July 2002, when the highly publicized WHI (Women's Health Initiative) study first reported that HRT (hormone replacement therapy) with an estrogen-progestin combination significantly increased breast cancer risk, particularly among women on such therapy for more than five years. Estrogen therapy alone did not show an increased risk of breast cancer.

Once the study was published, women and doctors quickly responded, and by the end of 2002, HRT use declined by almost 40 percent. That's more than twenty million *fewer* HRT prescriptions.

Given the link between certain kinds of HRT and breast cancer shown by the WHI study, combined with the dramatic drop in breast cancer rates once doctors stopped writing so many prescriptions for HRT, clearly there is some cause for concern for women considering such therapy. Any woman considering HRT should seriously weigh the risks and benefits of HRT to her health.

On a related note, oral contraceptives in premenopausal women do not appear to influence breast cancer risk later in life.

Deodorants/Antibiotics

If you haven't already received an alarmist e-mail about the supposed link between deodorant and breast cancer, your Internet connection must be down. There is, however, no conclusive link between breast cancer and deodorant/antiperspirant use.

The hypothesis is that substances in antiperspirants (such as parabens) may be absorbed through the skin in the underarm area, particularly when used in conjunction with shaving. However, a study of more than eight hundred women by researchers at the National Cancer Institute failed to show any link between deodorant/antiperspirant use and development of breast cancer.

A different study looked at breast cancer survivors and recorded patterns of antiperspirant use. While this appeared to show a younger age of diagnosis in women with more underarm cosmetic use, it provided no conclusive cause. My recommendation: don't change your personal hygiene habits because you're afraid of breast cancer.

Antibiotics also have been linked to breast cancer risk. A study funded by the NCI studied computer databases of more than two thousand women who had developed breast cancer and more than seven thousand women who had no personal history of breast cancer. They then compared how many days the women had used antibiotics over many years. Women who had used antibiotics for more than five hundred days in a seventeen-year period had twice the risk of breast cancer compared to women who had taken no antibiotics. This, of course, does not mean antibiotics cause breast cancer, only that their excessive use is associated with breast cancer.

Antibiotics are essential in fighting bacterial infections. Nevertheless, at least in the United States, they tend to be overused. Given the potential link between heavy antibiotic use and the development of breast cancer, women would be wise to use antibiotics judiciously and only when absolutely necessary.

The Great Uncontrollable: Genetics

We've spent most of this chapter talking about things you can control—what you eat, how much you weigh, how frequently you exercise, and what you put in and on your body. Now let's talk about what you can't control: who gave birth to you and all the hundreds of millions of lines of genetic coding that make *you*.

The majority of breast cancer is "sporadic," meaning it occurs randomly without a pattern in a family. About 5 to 7 percent of breast cancer is, however, "hereditary," meaning it is linked to a specific gene that can be passed down through families. The specific name of the genes important in hereditary breast cancer is BRCA genes (BReast CAncer genes).

Knowing your family's history of breast cancer is very important. This includes your father's family history of breast cancer as well (his mother and sisters, in particular). It is also not out of the question for men to develop breast cancer. When they do, it is typically genetic and therefore quite important for his daughters, nieces, and granddaughters to know about.

Women who have genetically linked breast cancer have special "features." They tend to develop breast cancer at an earlier age (less than fifty years) and may also have a family or personal history of ovarian cancer. They may have breast cancer that develops in both breasts. Some distinct populations of people have been found to collectively have a higher risk of developing hereditary breast cancer. These are called "founder" mutations, and an example would be Jewish women from Eastern Europe.

The importance of knowing your family history of breast cancer cannot be overstated. If you have a family history of breast cancer, it is critically important that you do what you can to reduce your risk, either through surveillance, surgery, or preventive medications. As much as some people would prefer it to be otherwise, you can't pick your family. And you can't undo the medical issues that have plagued them for generations.

Inflammatory Breast Cancer

There is an uncommon type of breast cancer that deserves to be singled out. *Inflammatory breast cancer* is a particularly deadly form and it presents in an unusual manner. Most breast cancer is found either on a screening mammogram or by feeling an abnormal lump during a breast examination. Inflammatory breast cancer, however, appears as **redness, swelling, and dimpling of the breast**. It commonly is mistaken for a breast infection and initially treated with antibiotics. Even more alarmingly, a mammogram often does not show a distinct mass. Therefore, women must be alert to the symptoms and request a breast biopsy or MRI scan if they show any symptoms of IBC.

Screening

The most important thing for every woman to know is that, regardless of her risk factors, regular screening is crucial. Screening is undertaken in an asymptomatic woman to find unsuspected breast cancer when it is small and while there is still a possibility of cure.

Yearly breast mammography remains the cornerstone of screening. There is universal agreement that annual mammographic screening reduces death from breast cancer by at least 50 percent.

Many of my patients don't have *any* risk factors for breast cancer. They're slim, healthy, eat the right things, don't drink much alcohol, and don't have a family history of the disease. Yet there they are, in my office.

What's the difference between the women who live and the women who die from the disease? Very frequently, it's screening. Regular screening can detect cancer when it is small and easier to combat.

Fortunately mammography techniques continue to improve. Digital mammograms use computer software to help read the mammogram; they are now widely available and may improve detection of breast cancer. Remember that while breast mammography is an excellent screening tool, it is not perfect. If you can feel a mass in your breast and a mammogram is unrevealing, it should be biopsied or imaged by an alternative method.

In May 2007, the American Cancer Society revised its screening guidelines for breast cancer. It recommended that higher-risk women, such as those with hereditary breast cancer or women with a lifetime risk of developing breast cancer greater than 20 percent, should have screening mammograms supplemented with MRI scans of the breast. More refining of these recommendations may occur in the future.

Despite the overwhelming evidence of the lifesaving abilities of regular screening, and the risks associated with not getting it done, many women continue to find excuses not to get a regular mammogram. I will tell you what I tell them: early detection saves lives, and regular mammograms are the first step in early detection. Don't make any more excuses. Get a friend and *go*.

RECOMMENDED RESOURCES

There is a wealth of resources for women looking to know more about breast cancer. Here are a few of the most reliable.

Internet:

> http://www.komen.org/
> http://www.cancer.gov/cancer_information/cancer_type/breast/

http://www.breastcancerfund.org
http://www.breastcancerdiy.com/
http://www.imaginis.com/
http://liv.com/
http://www.gloriagemma.org/

Books:

Dr. Susan Love's Breast Book by Dr. Susan Love

Breast Fitness: An Optimal Exercise and Health Plan for Reducing Your Risk of Breast Cancer by Dr. Anne McTiernan, Dr. Julie Gralow, and Lisa Talbott

Better Breast Health – for Life! by Tirza Derflinger, Deborah Breakell, Carrie Louise Daenell, and Carol Dalton

The Secret of Health: Breast Wisdom by Ben Johnson and Kathleen Barnes

The 10 Best Questions for Surviving Breast Cancer: The Script You Need to Take Control of Your Health by Dede Bonner and Marisa C. Weiss

Breast Cancer Survival Manual, Fourth Edition: A Step-by-Step Guide for the Woman with Newly Diagnosed Breast Cancer by John Link

Just Get Me Through This!: The Practical Guide to Breast Cancer by Deborah A. Cohen and Robert M. Gelfand, M.D.

Choices in Breast Cancer Treatment: Medical Specialists and Cancer Survivors Tell You What You Need to Know (A Johns Hopkins Press Health Book) by Kenneth D. Miller, M.D.

Breast Cancer: The Complete Guide: Fifth Edition by Acer Hirshaut, Peter Pressman, and Jane Brody

CHAPTER 13

WHAT'S SLEEP GOT TO DO WITH IT?

In bed, my real love has always been the sleep that rescued me by allowing me to dream.
—*Luigi Pirandello*

Thoughts from Mary Jo:

Have you ever tried to bake a cake and left out one of the ingredients? In baking, one small ingredient can make the difference between a superior cake and one that is a total flop. So it is with your health. You need every ingredient for success. If you learn nothing else from this book, it should be that for your health to be a success you have to have four ingredients:

1. Healthy eating habits
2. Regular movement
3. An optimistic attitude
4. Plenty of sleep

In chapter 9, I discussed how menopause interrupted my sleep. Without proper sleep, I made unhealthy food choices, was too tired to exercise, and was grumpy. I gained weight as a result.

There have been numerous studies on how much sleep we each need in order to be healthy. Dr. Sahni will give us the most up-to-date information.

Sweet dreams!

What the Doctor Has to Say: Jyotsna Sahni, M.D.

Sleep

I love my bed. I love my sheets and pillows. I love to sleep. But sleep wasn't always a joy for me. Like forty million Americans, I have had problems with sleep. We may not understand why we sleep, but we know we can't live without it. We spend one-third of our lives sleeping! Sleep is crucial to life. When we experience sleep problems, it can take a toll on the quality of our lives.

What Happens When We Sleep?

If you stop to think about it, sleep is kind of interesting. Studies observing people sleep while being attached to machines recording brain waves show that sleep is like a sine wave, gently undulating throughout the night.

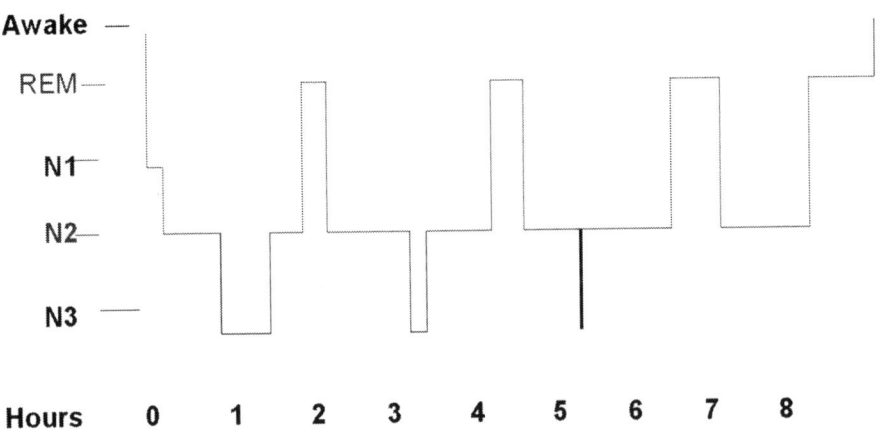

Known as "sleep architecture," sleep has four stages. Each cycle lasts roughly ninety minutes. Stages 1 and 2 are light, and if I call your name you'll wake right up. But stage 3 is deep and restorative.

We do a lot of work during this stage. For example, we make hormones, like growth hormone that keeps us young, testosterone that keeps us sexy, and thyroid hormone that keeps our metabolisms healthy. During deep sleep, we even make immune proteins that fight off infection and disease. Your mother was right when she warned that staying up too late and not getting enough sleep will make you sick. Now there's science to prove it.

After stages 1 through 3, we fall into REM sleep, which stands for "Rapid Eye Movement." This is our dream cycle, our lightest sleep. Our brains are very active during this stage of sleep. If I were Sigmund Freud, I'd say the dream cycle is where we do our emotional processing. He may have been right, but now we know the dream cycle helps our memory consolidation and processing speed. Everyone dreams, although not all of us remember our dreams. REM accounts for about 25 percent of our sleep.

Interestingly, we have a wake cycle just like we have a sleep cycle. This twenty-four-hour rhythm is called the Circadian rhythm. It is governed by nature's cycles of light and dark and day and night. This internal clock affects the production of hormones, our body temperature and heart rate, among other physiological processes. We tend to be most alert at ten o'clock in the morning and become increasingly tired as the day wears on, with one to four p.m. being an "afternoon lull." This is when most of America reaches for a Starbucks coffee and a candy bar. (If we lived in Spain or Mexico we would honor this dip in alertness and take a "siesta," or afternoon nap.) We feel more awake again from six to nine p.m. Most of us are programmed to sleep when it gets dark, so it's best to avoid driving between two and six a.m., when the urge to sleep is almost irresistible.

There are differences in our Circadian rhythms based on stage of life and also among individuals. For example, teenagers tend to like going to bed later and waking up late in the morning. They also need closer to nine hours of sleep, a little more than the typical adult. This tendency to sleep late and wake up late is known as "delayed phase disorder" and most of us outgrow this pattern eventually. Some people, often known as night people or "night owls," do not. Their rhythm simply prefers the night, when they are most alert and energetic. Conversely, some people find they are best in the morning; these folks are called morning people or "morning larks." Jokes about "early bird" dinners starting at four p.m. are often made about senior citizens. Many of us, as we age, prefer to go to bed earlier at night and wake up earlier in the morning. If bedtime has become unreasonably early (i.e., seven p.m.), then this is known as advanced phase disorder.

Circadian Rhythm

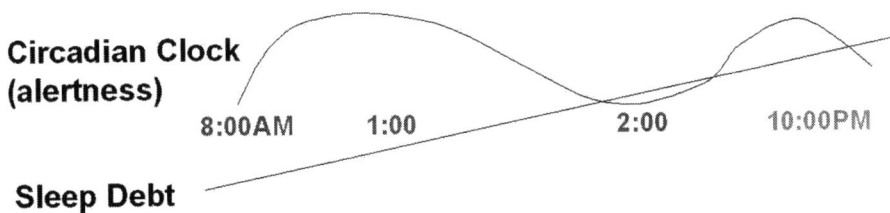

Circadian Clock (alertness)   8:00AM   1:00   2:00   10:00PM

Sleep Debt

How Much Sleep Do We Need?

The definition of "well rested" is the ability to stay awake in a darkened room in the middle of the day. In fact, it's not normal to:

- Fall asleep if reading quietly in the afternoon
- "Drift off" at afternoon meetings or while waiting at red lights
- Sleep on airplanes
- Fall asleep watching TV in the early evenings
- Sleep when you are a passenger in a car
- Need caffeine and open windows to drive two hours

When my patients tell me they are "great" sleepers and can fall asleep "the minute my head hits the pillow," I challenge them. I ask, "If I can eat my whole lunch in two minutes, am I a great eater or am I too hungry?" If you can sleep two hours later on the weekend than you do during the workweek, you surely are sleep deprived.

Hopefully, you are well rested. If not, you may be sleepy. While sleeplessness may not kill you, it does create a "disability." For example, after sixteen hours awake (or after only six hours of sleep) your alertness is equivalent to a blood alcohol concentration level of 0.05 percent. That's like drinking two beers. You are actually mentally and physically impaired when you are sleep deprived. Most people function best with between eight and nine hours of sleep each night; studies show that most adult bodies want eight hours and fifteen minutes of sleep. Of course, some people do well on less, others need more.

Unfortunately, about 75 percent of Americans are sleep deprived and simply don't get enough shut-eye. Some of the worst industrial accidents of the twentieth century were caused by sleep deprivation, such as the Exxon Valdez oil spill in Alaska in 1989. The Chernobyl accident and the space shuttle Challenger disaster are other examples of the devastating effect of sleep deprivation. Closer to home, fatigue is cited as the most common cause of fatal accidents in truckers. In fact, about 17 percent of Americans fall asleep at the wheel each year! According to the National Sleep Foundation, the direct and indirect impact of daytime sleepiness and sleep disorders on the national economy is estimated to be one hundred billion dollars annually. (Starbucks takes in about eight billion dollars a year helping people cope with their sleepiness.)

How much sleep you need also depends on your stage in life. For example, newborn babies sleep most of the day and night, teenagers need more than nine hours, and adults need between eight and nine hours. (Contrary to common myth, the need for sleep doesn't decline with age.)

Interestingly, one common consequence of sleep deprivation is hunger. In fact, some of the very same chemicals that control sleep also control hunger, such as cortisol (stress chemical), neuropeptide Y (carbohydrate hunger), hypocretin/orexin (narcolepsy), gallanin (fat hunger), and grehlin (acute hunger chemical). What this means is that we may reach for food because we are tired, not because we are actually hungry. Since these hormones overlap, the true cause of hunger may be masked. Sleep more, weigh less? Yes! Studies have suggested that people lose weight with increased sleep. Next time you reach for that jelly donut, ask yourself if what you really need is a good night's sleep!

Another consequence of sleep deprivation is increased pain. Some disorders like fibromyalgia or arthritis are characterized by pain, but are exacerbated by a lack of adequate sleep. Pain can make it hard to fall asleep and keep you up at night, but it can actually be made worse by poor sleep. This vicious cycle can keep you from healing. Sleep more, hurt less? Probably.

Sleep deprivation also leads to problems with functional cognitive abilities like memory, learning, and logical reasoning. Studies prove that people without good sleep make more mistakes, especially in tasks that require attentiveness, like driving a car or taking a test. In fact, students raise their grade point averages by getting more sleep.

Do Hormones Affect Sleep?

Of course they do! In women who menstruate, the first few days of a woman's period can make her sleep poorly because of menstrual cramps or bloating. During the week or two before a woman's period, the premenstrual or luteal phase, falling progesterone levels may make it more difficult to fall asleep and stay asleep. Some women feel extremely sleepy during the day and need more sleep than usual.

For pregnant women in the first trimester, nausea and breast tenderness may affect sleep, along with anxiety about being pregnant. In the second trimester, the fetus is growing and pushing on the bladder, making trips to the bathroom interrupt sleep. In the final trimester, women report the most trouble with sleep. At this time, they may experience heartburn, leg cramps, sinus congestion, frequent trips to the bathroom, difficulty breathing due to the fetus pushing against the diaphragm, and an inability to find a comfortable position.

Some things that may help pregnant women include sleeping on the left side in the third trimester, using special "pregnancy" pillows and mattresses, cutting off fluids early in the evening to reduce visits to the bathroom during the night, short naps throughout the day, eating small, frequent meals, avoiding spicy foods that may lead to heartburn, and gentle regular exercise that includes stretching to prevent muscle cramps.

Women who have never snored before may start in pregnancy because of a swelling of the nasal passages. If the snoring is severe enough to block nasal passages, obstructive sleep apnea may result, leading to non-restorative sleep, high blood pressure, and a diminished supply of oxygen to the fetus. This serious condition can hurt both the mother and the unborn baby.

Fifteen percent of women in the third trimester will develop restless leg syndrome (described below). This is usually a result of deficiency of iron and/or folate. Fortunately, this annoying condition usually resolves postpartum.

Even after the baby is born, a new mother's sleep is often disturbed because she must feed her baby frequently throughout the night. This fragmented sleep schedule can contribute to "postpartum blues" or, worse, to full-blown postpartum depression. Sleeping when the new baby sleeps may help a woman catch up on lost sleep; also, having good child care and household support may improve the situation.

I spoke briefly about sleep disturbance in menopause in chapter 9. Sleep disturbance in menopause is very common. Hot flashes and night sweats can interrupt quality sleep. Drops in estrogen may lead to waking every ninety minutes, which then interrupts both quantity and quality of sleep. Drops in progesterone affect the drive to breathe, making snoring and sleep apnea more common in women after menopause. Being aware of these changes, treating them appropriately, and especially being rigorous about good sleep hygiene during menopause are all important for mood, memory, energy, and overall good health.

Insomnia

"Doctor, I can't sleep!" One of the most common complaints I hear from my patients is trouble sleeping. Insomnia means that you can't sleep. There are two main kinds of insomnia. The first is when a patient tells me she simply can't fall asleep, or that it takes too unreasonably long to do so. The average person takes five to twenty minutes to fall asleep. This is normal. But if it takes a lot longer to fall asleep, there could be a problem. This is called sleep onset insomnia; the onset of sleep is delayed. Conversely, sometimes a patient has no trouble falling asleep, but has difficulty staying asleep. This is called sleep maintenance insomnia. Some patients, unfortunately, suffer from both types of insomnia. Women, more than men, have trouble with insomnia in general.

There are multiple reasons for both types of insomnia. I have outlined many below and how to handle them.

Many **medications**, both over-the-counter and prescribed, can affect sleep. The treatment is to avoid these drugs, use them sparingly, or find better substitutes if possible. Here is a list of common drugs that keep people awake:

- Alcohol
- Nicotine
- Cocaine
- Caffeine
- Decongestants like Sudafed

- Ritalin, diet pills, or other stimulants
- Ginkgo and other herbals
- Ephedrine
- Beta-blockers
- Albuterol for asthma; theophylline for COPD
- Wellbutrin, Prozac, and many other antidepressants
- Prednisone and other steroids
- Many more

Insomnia is typically a symptom, not a problem. By working on the problem, we can usually treat the insomnia. The behavioral treatment for insomnia has proven benefit; it's actually better than drugs in many cases. These suggestions for good "sleep hygiene" may seem obvious, but you'd be surprised how well they work!

Avoid Caffeine

Caffeine is found in coffee, tea, cola, diet pills, Excedrin, and even chocolate. A new study led by researchers at the University of Toronto found that people with mutations in one or both genes responsible for breaking down caffeine will break it down up to four times more slowly than people with a normal gene. The slower your body breaks it down, the longer the stimulating effect. Also, individuals with the slow version of the gene have an increased risk of heart disease from as little as two cups of coffee a day.

The study also found that those under fifty who had fast versions of the gene actually had less heart disease when they drank one to three cups a day. Only through genetic testing can you find out which genes you have. Typically, the half-life of caffeine is seven hours. This means that the liver clears half the caffeine you have in your body in seven hours. What this means is that for some people caffeine stays in the system for a ridiculously long time. For example, if you drink four cups of coffee in the morning, you may literally go to bed with one in you at night. Regardless of genes, too much caffeine can cause jitteriness, palpitations, and anxiety. If you have trouble sleeping, eliminating caffeine is an important first step to good sleep. But decaffeinate yourself slowly; caffeine is addictive, and stopping cold turkey will often bring on a wicked caffeine withdrawal headache that may last for days.

Avoid Nicotine

Nicotine, found in cigarettes and chewing tobacco, is a stimulant like caffeine, and can keep you awake. I'm sure you know the other serious health consequences of smoking. You should avoid it at all costs.

Avoid Alcohol

While alcohol initially makes you sleepy, as your body clears it from your system you can develop a restless sleep, night sweats, and headaches. To help reduce these effects, keep in mind my three rules for alcohol and sleep. The first is obvious: "less is better." The less you drink, the fewer bad effects on your sleep. The second rule is "earlier is better." This way, you have more time to clear the drink while you are still awake, and the less it will affect your sleep. Finally, the third rule is "with food is better." Food slows the absorption of alcohol; it won't hit you as hard and you'll be less drunk. For every drink, it takes your liver about two hours to clear it. For example, you need two hours to clear one drink, four hours to clear two drinks, and six hours to clear three drinks. Also, try to drink one glass of water for every alcoholic beverage you consume. (Another reason to go light on the sauce: more than one drink a day for women increases their risk for breast cancer! One drink is defined as five ounces of wine, twelve ounces of beer, or one and one-half ounces of hard liquor.)

Get Exercise

Exercise is good for you for a million reasons, as Mary Jo and Lu have outlined in chapter 4; it even helps relieve stress and encourages good sleep. But for some people, exercise is so energizing that it makes it hard to fall sleep. If you get too revved up by exercise, give yourself at least three hours between working out and bedtime.

Eat Right

Don't go to bed hungry or stuffed from a large meal. Both can interrupt your sleep. Some foods may help promote sleep, like milk, eggs, potatoes, bananas, peaches, walnuts, apricots, oats, asparagus, almonds, pumpkin, artichokes, tuna, and halibut. Avoid sugary foods before bed because they can make you overly stimulated. Cut off fluids after eight p.m. so you don't have to interrupt sleep time with bathroom breaks.

A Good Sleep Environment

Build yourself a cocoon. **Stay in the dark**! Get light-blocking blinds; use a drape clip or an eye mask or both. The light from a night-light, digital clock, a streetlight, or even moonlight coming through a crack in the blinds can interrupt your sleep. Also, avoid bright light before bedtime. If you get up during the night to use the bathroom, try to use only a low-illumination night-light to guide you, rather than bright overhead lights.

Keep it quiet. Again, noise from traffic, a TV blaring in the next room, a dog barking, or someone snoring next to you can interrupt sleep. Earplugs are inexpensive and available at drugstores everywhere. Carpeting and drapes in the bedroom may absorb sound. You also may want to keep a fan on or invest in a "white noise" machine to mask ambient noises.

Finally, **keep it cool** at night (another reason for the fan to be on!). The best temperature for sleep is 68–72 degrees Fahrenheit. Temperatures warmer than 75 degrees or cooler than 54 degrees will disrupt sleep. We feel sleepy any time our body temperature drops, which it does in the afternoon and then again at night. This is why we feel sleepy at these times. Our body temperature falls to its lowest points at about four hours into our night's sleep.

Nap Smart

Sometimes, a quick power nap early in the day is wonderfully refreshing. But if you sleep more than half an hour, you will wake up groggy and it will take longer to get going again. Also, if you sleep too long, you may find yourself staring at the ceiling at night. Limit your nap to twenty minutes.

Save the Bed

Save the bed for only sleep (and for sex!). Create a conditioned response to your bed. When you see it, your body should have the following unconscious conversation: "Ahhh! I love my bed; this is where I love to sleep. My bed is my source of rest, comfort, and intimacy. My eyelids are getting heavy..." Instead, many people regard their beds as a place to watch TV, read the paper, work on their laptops, eat, etc. Some people get anxious when they think about going to bed because they are worried they'll have another restless night. This is a form of "performance anxiety."

I am asking you, for the sake of good sleep, to change your habits. This means doing a feng shui thing to your bedroom. Make it clean, uncluttered. Use calming colors like blues, greens, and earth tones. Get rid of the TV from your bedroom. Save violent, dramatic TV and movies for daytime; those disturbing images can influence our ability to fall asleep and the content of our dreams. Even kick out the pets! Pets may sleep in their own doggy or kitty beds in your bedroom, but not in your bed itself. Children (when appropriate) also should be encouraged to sleep in their own beds and rooms. Sometimes partners snore or jerk around in bed, or otherwise disturb your sleep. Keep channels of communication open and find solutions together to help quality of sleep for both of you. Create a peaceful, pleasant environment that is conducive to good sleep.

Have a Sleep Ritual

This is the part of good sleep habits that leads to good sleep. Little children are conditioned by their parents to drift off into slumber by having a sleep ritual: now it's time to brush the teeth, now it's time to wear the pajamas, now it's time to read the story, now it's time to turn off the light. "Good night, moon" also means good night to little Sally or Jim. Adults with sleep problems need to get back to the basics, too. Go to bed at the same and wake up at the same time—regardless of whether it is Saturday, Sunday, or a holiday.

Thirty to sixty minutes before bedtime, roam around your home and turn off extraneous lights, check that the doors are locked. Take a warm bath. Use "grounding" scents like lavender, vanilla, or cloves. Rub your feet with sesame oil. Maybe listen to a relaxation CD or have a small (three ounces) cup of chamomile tea or boiled milk with a pinch of cardamom. Do some deep breathing. Say your prayers. Climb into bed with your earplugs and eye mask and wait for sleep to come to you. You can't make yourself fall asleep; all you can do is make the environment conducive for sleep.

A Good Bed

A good bed that is not too old or lumpy and that is appropriately soft, hard, thin, thick, etc., is necessary for good sleep, too. The bed also should be spacious enough so everyone involved can stretch out comfortably. Pillows should support the head and be free of dust mites and fungal spores that lead to allergies and asthma. Many of my patients complain of waking up with a stuffy nose or puffy eyes; I ask, "When was the last time you replaced your pillow?" Interestingly, synthetic pillows seem to hold more bacteria and dust mite fecal material than do feather pillows.

Stimulus Control/Sleep Restriction

This is another sleep-promoting technique for sleep onset insomnia. Since our goal is to build a positive association with your bed and a good night's sleep, if you can't fall asleep after thirty minutes, get out of bed. Don't stay in bed tossing and turning. Get up and involve yourself in a relaxing activity, such as listening to soothing music or reading a boring book, until you feel sleepy. You don't want to do anything interesting that may keep you up. Read the dictionary rather than a gripping mystery novel. You also don't want to be productive because you don't want any positive association to be built around your insomnia. Therefore, don't clean the kitchen or balance your checkbook. Simply engage in a boring activity until you feel sleepy again and then go back to bed. If you still can't fall asleep within thirty more minutes, get up again and repeat the whole process. The idea is not to spend nine hours in bed, when you only sleep for six.

When you are in bed, you should either be asleep or about to fall asleep. You should get to bed at the same time each night and get up at the same time every morning. Avoid naps during this conditioning process, even if you're sleepy. If you sleep during the day, you are less tired at night. It's okay for a day or two to walk around tired while you build new associations. You are more likely to sleep at night in your bed like you're supposed to if you are tired when you get there.

Don't Look at the Clock

Looking at the clock will just give you anxiety. Cover it up or remove it from the bedroom.

Here are many of the sleep issues my patients ask me about.

Anxiety and Sleep

Often, worry and anxiety can make it difficult for us to sleep well. A mind-body technique like meditation can help calm the mind. (For some specific techniques, see chapter 15.) The Art of Living course teaches a simple yogic breathing technique that cured my busy, anxious mind. Now I sleep better than ever! Sometimes, a good therapist may be necessary to help you "think" about things differently, or teach you biofeedback or progressive relaxation exercises.

Sometimes, a simple journaling technique can be helpful. Keep a pen and paper next to the bed, jot down a few key words of what's bothering you, and then rest assured that anything you have to worry about will be there in the morning. Tell yourself, "I can sleep now. This problem is on paper now. I won't forget about it. In the morning, I will deal with it." This way, you talk yourself into letting go of the worry until morning, when you can actually do something about it. This inner dialogue can soothe you; you give yourself permission to fall asleep. Needless to say, if you have anxiety, you must avoid caffeine and other stimulants. You are stimulated enough by the thoughts in your head; caffeine will just make things worse. If anxiety is more than mild and occasional, you should speak to your doctor and get professional help.

Depression and Sleep

Depression is about two or three times more common in women than men. While everybody has a down day, depression is much more than that and deserves to be diagnosed and treated like any other medical condition. It is a serious condition and can result in death. Having said that, it's interesting to note that sad mood, irritability, difficulty making decisions, and a sense of hopelessness and helplessness can be part of a diagnosis of clinical depression, and the same exact symptoms may occur in sleep deprivation. Insomnia itself can even cause depression. Early morning awakening can signal it. Depression isn't something to underplay or deny. You need to seek professional help; speak with your doctor. Fortunately, depression (and sleep deprivation) is extremely treatable, if not curable! (For details on depression, see chapter 3.)

Pain and Sleep

As a routine part of my evaluation for sleep problems, I now ask the very important question, "Does anything hurt?" Headaches, arthritis, and heartburn are more common in women than men. Pain can make it hard to fall asleep and stay asleep. Like depression, it's usually treatable. You don't have to suffer from most pain.

Appropriate treatment with supplements, medications, and therapies targeted at the cause of pain can be employed to reduce it and maximize good sleep.

Bladder Problems and Sleep

Many patients tell me they have to get up several times during the night to use the bathroom and that this is why they have poor sleep. I doubt it. While it's a common complaint, I think it's usually a misperception. As adults, we are designed to hold it for eight hours. There are exceptions to this. For example, you may have multiple sclerosis and a "neurogenic" bladder, or another clear issue of incontinence. Also, if you drank a gallon of water before going to bed, of course you'll have to get up during the night to release it. If you drank a gallon of iced tea it would be even worse, because the caffeine would act as a stimulant and also a mild diuretic. The solution to this is simple: cut off fluids early in the evening.

Another cause of nighttime urination is a urinary tract infection, which may cause urinary frequency, urgency, and burning. Also, taking a diuretic before bed, such HCTZ or Lasix for blood pressure or heart issues, or drinking a diuretic "dieter's" tea such as dandelion root, would be very understandable reasons to rise during the night. But again, these are exceptions to the rule. Most of the time people wake up for whatever reason, notice they have a little pressure on the bladder, and get up and use the bathroom. I ask my patients, "Do you pass a lot of urine when you get up during the night?" The answer is overwhelmingly, "No." We think we're getting up to urinate, when in fact we're awake for another reason. If we correct that other reason, we'll be mostly okay with the nighttime urination.

Why "mostly" okay? Because we get ourselves into a habit, and habits are hard to break. You may actually have to talk yourself out of making that trip to the bathroom. Say to yourself, "It's okay to be awake for a moment during the night. I don't really have to go to the bathroom." Then turn over, take a few deep breaths, and let yourself fall back to sleep. I allow my patients to wake up once or possibly twice during the night to use the bathroom, if they can fall right back to sleep and the trip does not get in the way of their quantity and quality of sleep. If it's more often, we should do something about it.

There are some medical reasons for poor sleep that won't respond to behavioral treatments alone. These include obstructive sleep apnea, periodic limb movement disorder, restless leg syndrome, narcolepsy, and nocturnal eating disorder.

Obstructive Sleep Apnea (OSA)

OSA is a disorder characterized by breathing that temporarily stops during sleep. To make the official diagnosis, you must hold your breath ("apnea") for at least ten seconds five times in one hour of sleep. While you hold your breath, levels of carbon dioxide, which your body considers an acid, rise in your blood. When your blood gets too acidic, your body wakes you up and you start to breathe again to blow off the carbon dioxide. Then you fall back to sleep, hold your breath again, and the cycle continues. You may not realize that you're waking up or you may awaken with a "resuscitative" snort.

About 5 percent of the population has OSA; that's roughly the same as the number of people who have asthma. We may have heard of asthma, but most of us are ignorant of OSA. Most of the time, it's easy to identify and to treat. The number-one symptom is excessive daytime sleepiness. Patients with OSA fall asleep at inappropriate times, such as in a business meeting or at a red light, or even while driving! These patients tend to snore loudly. The snoring is a result of a partial narrowing of the soft tissues of the nasal and oral passages caused by large tonsils and adenoids, poor muscle tone, a long, soft palate, and/or limp tissue. Many apneic patients are overweight. Like body weight, snoring tends to increase as we age, especially in women after menopause.

What factors may promote sleep apnea?

- Large neck (>17" men, >16" women)
- Small chin
- Family history
- Men more than women before menopause
- Women after menopause
- Stuffy and narrow nose
- Alcohol/sedating drugs

People with OSA are at higher risk for high blood pressure, heart attacks, arrhythmias, and motor vehicle accidents.

We test for OSA by taking a good history of the patient's sleepiness and snoring, examining the patient for being overweight, having a small chin, large tonsils, etc., and by doing a "sleep study." This entails an overnight stay at a hospital or sleep lab, where a patient can be observed asleep while wearing probes that will monitor breathing, heartbeats, brain waves, and leg movement.

Treatment for sleep apnea may include simple things, such as choosing to sleep on the side rather than the back, and avoiding alcohol or sleeping pills that may relax tissues in the nose and oral cavity. In addition, treating a stuffy nose by using nasal irrigation, nasal steroids, or decongestants to help reduce swelling may be effective in reducing snoring and apnea. Sometimes simple interventions are not enough. CPAP ("continuous positive airway pressure") is a breathing machine the patient wears during the night that blows air into the nose and/or oral cavity to keep the soft tissues from collapsing. A dental device that pulls the jaw forward can keep the passages open for good airflow. Finally, as a last resort, people may opt for surgery to correct anatomical flaws that contribute to a narrow airway, such as large tonsils and adenoids.

Periodic Leg Movement Disorder

Periodic leg movement disorder is a disorder in which the legs (and occasionally the arms) twitch during the night, causing a brief awakening. The twitching typically occurs every twenty to forty seconds and lasts between half a second to five seconds. The kicks can involve the big toe, ankle, knee, or even the hip. They can occur in one leg, both, or alternate. Since the kicks usually occur during light sleep, stages 1 and 2, it may be difficult to fall asleep. Some patients are unaware of their kicking but know they have trouble falling asleep; others feel that their feet are extremely cold; some report excessive daytime sleepiness. Bed partners are often very aware of the kicking behavior and may sleep elsewhere to avoid being kicked all night. The diagnosis is made by a sleep study and is defined by five or more kicks in each hour of sleep that cause an awakening. The underlying cause of periodic leg movement disorder is not well understood, but it does seem to have a genetic component and gets worse with advancing age. Some medications exacerbate it while others may help manage this condition.

Restless Leg Syndrome

Restless leg syndrome is a disorder characterized by an uncomfortable creeping or crawling feeling in the legs, feet, or thighs that is temporarily relieved by movement. Sometimes patients describe "pins and needles" feelings and try to rub their legs or walk it off to relieve the discomfort. It can make falling asleep and staying asleep difficult. It can also occur during the day when a woman has to sit still at her desk or in a movie. Restless leg syndrome is thought to be due to a low dopamine level in the brain. It is about 60 percent genetic and occurs more in women than men. It is more commonly seen in kidney failure, rheumatoid arthritis, and during pregnancy. Caffeine and other drugs, fatigue, and extreme temperatures of either hot or cold can exacerbate this condition. It tends to begin in the third decade of life and get worse over time. Patients with restless leg syndrome often have periodic limb movements, too. Fortunately, along with several new effective drugs, adequate doses of iron may help treat it and give relief to the patients who suffer from it.

Narcolepsy

Narcolepsy is a rare chronic neurological disorder that occurs in about one in two thousand people. It's defined by a classic syndrome of four unusual symptoms. The first symptom is that patients with this disease have an irresistible urge to sleep during the day, called "sleep attacks." Next, 70 percent of patients may suddenly lose muscle tone or strength ("cataplexy"), especially following a strong emotional response to a funny joke or shocking news, for instance. "Hypnogogic hallucinations" are seen in 50 to 70 percent of patients; these are characterized by vivid visual and auditory dreamlike phenomena that often provoke fear and anxiety. Forty to 65 percent of patients experience "sleep paralysis." This may occur at the same time as the hypnogogic hallucinations, as the narcoleptic patient falls off to sleep. Her body is paralyzed except for eye movements and respirations. The onset of narcolepsy is typically in the teenage years or young adulthood and has a strong genetic component. Narcolepsy is considered a disorder of REM sleep. Periodic leg movement disorder is more common in patients with narcolepsy. Treatment today is very promising, with a combination of stimulants to fight daytime sleepiness and special sleeping pills to promote good nighttime sleep.

Nocturnal Sleep Eating Disorder

People with this rare disorder eat food during the night while they are seemingly asleep. They may not remember their behaviors in the morning because the parts of their brains that control memory are asleep. More than 65 percent of sufferers are women. Eating at night may be due to high levels of ghrelin, an acute hunger chemical, in the first hours of sleep. Some medications, like Ambien, can actually precipitate this condition.

Tooth Grinding

Tooth grinding, or "bruxism," is more common in children, tends to get better into adulthood, and runs in families. It typically occurs during stage 2 sleep and may disturb it. Bruxism may be made worse by anxiety and poor alignment of teeth and jaw. Sometimes the patient wakes up with a sore jaw, but most people are unaware that they grind their teeth. Often a bed partner reports hearing the grinding sound or a dentist comments on worn-down teeth. A dental device, in combination with relaxation techniques, can help.

Shift Workers

According to the National Sleep Foundation, 17 percent of Americans are shift workers. As a group, they tend to be more sleep deprived than people working a traditional "nine to five" job. It's hard to reset our internal circadian clocks. Our body's urge to sleep is strongest between midnight and six a.m. This is why 10 to 20 percent of shift workers report falling asleep on the job, especially on the second half of the shift. This also accounts for why it may be hard for shift workers to sleep during the day (their "night") despite being tired.

More health problems are likely for anyone who is sleep deprived, and the problems seem to be compounded for shift workers. For example, they experience more stomach problems (especially heartburn and indigestion), colds, flu, and weight gain than day workers. Female shift workers also suffer irregular menstrual cycles, difficulty getting pregnant, higher rates of miscarriages, premature births, and low-birth-weight babies. Even heart problems and higher blood pressure are more common. The risk of workplace accidents and automobile crashes rises for tired shift workers, especially on the drive to and from work. The tenets of good sleep hygiene as describe above are even more important for shift workers.

Jet Lag

I travel a lot, and so do my patients. While it's fun to travel and see the world, changing time zones can be tough on sleep. This conflict with your own internal clock and that of your travel location is known as "jet lag." A few days before you travel, try to gradually shift your sleep and wake times to those of your destination. When you get to your destination, adopt the prevailing sleep/wake time as soon as you can. In the morning, get some natural light in your eyes to send messages to the pineal gland, the part of your brain that makes melatonin. This will help reset your internal clock. In general, it is easier for us to travel east to west because this lengthens our days. While I am not a big proponent of drugs, in the case of jet lag, either an over-the-counter or prescribed sleep aid can be especially helpful. If you travel west to east, melatonin supplements may make it easier to fall asleep earlier than you are used to. This is because melatonin tricks your brain into thinking it's dark, and therefore time to go to sleep. Conversely, if you travel east to west, taking Benadryl, which tends to prolong the night and lets you sleep longer, is a better choice. To make the transition as smooth as possible, be staunch about avoiding caffeine and alcohol when you are jet-lagged.

When to Consult Your Doctor

When sleep problems are affecting the quality of your life for more than just a few days, it makes sense to speak with your doctor. While there are many things you can do to help yourself, sometimes we need more. You may benefit from a sleeping pill or pain pill for a short time while you get other things together. You may talk with your doctor to change your current prescription to make it more sleep-friendly. Sometimes a sleep study is necessary to diagnose sleep apnea, narcolepsy, periodic leg movement disorder, etc. Unfortunately, many regular doctors are uninformed about sleep issues; if yours can't help you, ask for a referral to a specialist. A good night's sleep can make you feel like you're on top of the world. You deserve to be there!

RECOMMENDED RESOURCES:

National Osteoporosis Foundation (NOF) is the nation's leading voluntary health organization solely dedicated to osteoporosis and bone health.
www.nof.org

Calcium Supplementation in Clinical Practice: A Review of Forms, Doses, and Indications. Straub, Deborah. *Nutrition in Clinical Practice* 22: 286-296, June 2007.

Effect of Selective Serotonin Reuptake Inhibitors on the Risk of Fracture. J. Brent Richards; Alexandra Papaioannou; Jonathan D. Adachi; Lawrence Joseph; Heather E. Whitson; Jerilynn C. Prior; David Goltzman; for the Canadian Multicentre Osteoporosis Study (CaMos) Research Group. *Arch Intern Med.* 2007; 167:188-194.

All I Want Is a Good Night's Sleep by Sonia Ancoli-Israel

National Sleep Foundation (NSF) is an independent nonprofit organization dedicated to improving public health and safety by achieving understanding of sleep and sleep disorders, and by supporting sleep-related education, research, and advocacy.
www.sleepfoundation.org

Power Sleep by Dr. James B. Maas

Thanks to Phil Eichling, M.D., (Canyon Ranch) for the wealth of information he has shared with me.

PART FIVE

YOU ARE WHAT YOU THINK: THE MIND-BODY CONNECTION

CHAPTER 14

THE HEART AND SOUL OF ANY WOMAN: Relationships

Thoughts from Mary Jo:

It will come as no shock to you that scientists have come to the conclusion that men and women are different. Imagine that! New research shows that men's and women's brains are different starting after eight weeks in utero.[11]

Something we have known all our lives is that female brains make more connections in areas that govern communications and emotions. The male brain makes more connections in areas that govern sex and aggression.[12] In other words, women are more relationship-oriented.

So what does that mean for us in our quest for a healthier and happier life? Most certainly for women (and probably for men as well), our relationships must be healthy and in balance for us to feel healthy and happy. Finding that place of balance is the key.

As a family law attorney for almost thirty years, I see what happens to women when their relationship with their spouse is in a state of imbalance. Especially when their relationship with their spouse is going poorly, it is very hard for women to continue to work on the other aspects of their health, i.e., exercise, nutrition, and spiritual life. For women, when that part of our life is not working, it's like one of the wheels has come off the cart and we have to drag it behind us.

As women, in order to have happiness, health, and harmony, we must continually work on our relationships and, when they break down, find methods to keep going on all four wheels.

"Happy women know that their worth is not determined by what they have or how they look, but rather by successful relationships and emotional well-being."[13]

Here are a few tips for successful relationships.

1. You and Your Spouse or Significant Other

Until recently, most marriages in the United States ended with the death of one of the partners, but divorce is now the number-one reason a marriage terminates. According to the U.S. Census Bureau, the national divorce ratio is one divorce for every two marriages. Because almost everyone is likely to be touched by divorce (whether directly or indirectly), it is important for us to understand how to prevent it.

A research team of psychologists and lawyers developed the conclusions discussed in the article written by my husband and I entitled "Divorce: Prevention, Survival, & Recovery." The team interviewed 169 attorneys, 126 mental health professionals, and seven ministers about the effects of divorce and coping skills for individuals going through a divorce.

Divorce Prevention

Do you want to live longer, healthier, wealthier, and sexier? *Stay married.* Studies show that married people live longer, suffer fewer health ailments, have a higher net worth, and enjoy more sex than single people. To stay married, couples need to focus on marital enrichment and, should the need arise, marital restoration.

A. Marital or "Significant Other" Enrichment

Communicate

Honest, open, and frequent communication is essential in marriage. Focus on friendship and partnership. Ask how your spouse is doing. After you ask, *listen* to the response. Acknowledge that you and your spouse may have different styles and purposes when communicating. Learn what those are so that you respond appropriately. Communication is the fuel you need to cruise love's highway and, like all fuel, it comes in different grades. The premium fuel that will keep your marriage in good condition for the long haul is *meaningful* communication.

Meaningful communication is heartfelt, nonjudgmental, and rigorously honest when necessary. It is initiated at random times as well as special times, and not just on your anniversary or right before sex. It frequently consists of an unmotivated, voluntary, and selfless act or statement, which makes your spouse feel special, loved, and appreciated. It can appear to others as a kind of secret code language that only lovers know. Think about how much it means to you when your spouse cooks your favorite dinner as a surprise, or leaves an unexpected love note in your briefcase that you open at the office, or a spontaneous pause on the way to dinner to say how wonderful you are. This kind of very personal, selfless communication of caring is soul food for your partner.

Flexibility and Adaptation

In all areas of marital enrichment, there is a common thread: flexibility and adaptation. People's values and goals evolve, but perhaps at different rates or in different directions. It is up to you to find a way to make these goals and values work together. For example, your sexual needs might change. Both partners have an obligation to keep an open mind and meet each other's expectations. You may desire a career change that requires flexibility in financial, time, or geographic expectations. One or both partners must adapt to these changes. As another example, you may hate horror movies, but occasionally you should sit through one if your spouse loves a good *Friday the 13th* flick. Flexibility and adaptation enable partners to continuously meet each other's changing needs.

Gender Roles

When you were dating, you may have been looking for a "man that fits the plan." By this, I mean that you had an expectation of how your significant other was going to fill a particular role. Early in life, some women have an expectation that they will work in the home to raise a family, while others see themselves in a corporate setting. Some men see themselves as the sole provider and protector and other men have an egalitarian view of marriage. Because of the evolution of values, circumstances, and goals during marriage, you need to be flexible in your expectations of gender roles. Equally important, be certain to accurately communicate these expectations to your spouse.

Time and Attention

Communicate to your significant other that the time and attention he or she gave you yesterday affects the quality (or occasion) of sex tonight. It's true—most women are often more expressive physically when they are satisfied emotionally. Such fulfillment comes from long-term satisfaction with the amount *and* quality of time and attention she receives. Women, this truism may also apply to you. People of both genders are more responsive when they are fulfilled.

So many couples complain that they don't have time. Make time. Make time to be together and time to be apart. Spend your together time together nurturing and displaying affection and communicating from the heart. Do simple things. Spend some of this time on "everyday" days—not just on anniversaries or birthdays.

Avoid Relationship Toxins

Relationship toxins are drugs, alcohol abuse, affairs, or violence. When one partner engages in these risky behaviors, it hurts both, and possibly the children as well. Risky behaviors cause irreparable damage; do not even "taste" a relationship toxin.

Never Stop Dating

During courtship, you probably felt special, cared for, and in love. Of course, everyone wants these things, so why stop the behaviors that generate these feelings? Make a date, hold a door, and give a hug. Never stop showing you care, and never stop dating your spouse. Remember a time in your courtship when you took a picnic in the park with just a blanket, some food, and a bottle of wine? Why not re-create that sweet moment, even if it's twenty years later? My husband and I have a date night every Friday and go to a movie. So that we don't have a disagreement about what movie to see, we go to the first one playing at the theater nearby after we both get home from work. We have seen some pretty good movies that way that we might not have seen otherwise. As long as one of us wants to stay, we stay. I look forward to Friday night because it is always a surprise.

Partner and Personal Passions

Although opposites may attract, studies show that people who are similar are more likely to stay together. To bridge a gap of differences, determine a passion and explore it together: art, yoga, running, baseball, or whatever you both love. By the same token, have a passion that you can enjoy on your own, to establish independent satisfaction. A motivating career is a common personal passion, but it can be many things.

Realistic Expectations

Expect "ever after" but know it's not easy to get there. Do not expect that you can change your partner or that your partner will remain the same forever. Frame and reframe positively. When life turns out differently than you expect, do not blame your spouse. Instead, work together to make a better reality.

Work

By now, you may have noticed that marital enrichment requires plenty of time and energy—actual work. You have to work to be fun, work to keep the romance alive, and work to meet expectations. It's not easy to remain flexible, adapt, and reframe expectations, but if you want a lasting marriage, this is what it takes!

"How'm I Doin', Honey?"

People need feedback to improve. At the office, you may have an annual review; in school, report cards come out every few months. Why not take inventory of your relationship periodically to communicate achievement, appreciation, and an agenda? You can make this a fun and nurturing event instead of a formal or threatening one. Every once in awhile, casually ask, "How'm I doin', honey?" Make a commitment that, when one partner asks this question, you both answer it honestly and lovingly. Make a pact to have an annual date weekend to a beach city, the mountains, or skiing, when you both agree to focus on enjoying the relationship and communicating about its progress.

B. Marital Restoration

When marital problems arise, accept responsibility for finding solutions without focusing on blame. Positive change requires effort by both spouses, but consider a neutral facilitator (such as a financial counselor, marital therapist, or life coach) to provide direction. A 2005 meta-analysis concluded that marital therapy or intervention produces positive results, whether the focus is on emotional improvements, behavioral improvements, or both.

Communication Problems

Many couples complain of conflict or disconnectedness in their communication—the root of divorce. Communication problems include the absence of openness, honesty, and bilateral interaction, as well as impaired ability to interpret communication. If communication has been neglected, address this immediately. Communication is the number-one area where marital counseling professionals can benefit couples as a neutral facilitator and educator. Although your efforts to communicate must never cease, such therapy typically requires only ten to twenty-six sessions.

Sexual Needs

The common root of unmet sexual need is unmet expectation. Typically, an unmet sexual expectation occurs because a certain sexual behavior or relationship existed prior to or early in a marriage, and later in the marriage one spouse loses interest in the same behavior or relationship. Because the other spouse expects the same sexual behavior or relationship, he or she becomes frustrated and feels rejected, perpetuating communication breakdown. The rejected spouse may turn to risky behavior alternatives, such as affairs.

When sexual needs are not met, address them honestly and lovingly, but frankly. Be willing to remain emotionally flexible. Sexual relationships do evolve, but if you think yours will dissolve, seek a qualified sexual "rediscovery" course or counselor. Just as you should continue communicating lovingly, you should continue expressing your love physically, enjoying anticipation and striving to have sex that is not "routine."

The Many Faces of Money

Money has many faces. Of course, you can have too little, the discomfort of which may cause daily stresses that can lead to marital problems. Then you can actually have too much money, and if perspectives are unhealthy, money can become more important than people. Even worse is when partners have a disparate amount of or access to money. Money is a kind of power, so an imbalance of money creates an imbalance of power.

The bottom line is that partners must accept that a healthy relationship is not based on how much money one or the other brings to the table.

Couples fight about money they have or do not have and what they do or do not do with that money. When you disagree on how to allocate income, seek professional advice from a financial counselor or an online personal finance program to take some of the positioning out of the allocation decision. Again, putting a neutral professional's advice between your positions bridges the path to solution.[14]

2. Co-Workers

We spend more than half of our waking hours in the workplace, and yet we spend very little time cultivating relationships with our co-workers. I am not saying your co-workers need to be your friends, although they can be. What I am saying is that your relationships with your co-workers are extremely important to your overall well-being. Additionally, our professional success is not just tied to how well we perform our jobs, but also to how well we get along with others in the workplace.

Try to become aware of your persona in the workplace. Pick two or three people and ask them to speak honestly about how you are perceived. Ask if you are considered a team player. Ask if you let your personal life interfere with your attitude at work. Promise these people that you are not going to be angry with any of their comments. Above all, LISTEN!

Next, take the information you have learned and make an action plan of how you can improve relationships. For example, if one of the things you were told is that you don't listen, for the next day have a plan to actively listen. After you have done it for one day, then do it for two and three. See if you can make it a habit. Another example would be, "You criticize too much." Make it your goal for a week not to criticize.

You aren't going to be perfect, but you will be more aware of your faults and shortcomings and can slowly begin to change them.

3. Friends

Indeed, we do not really live unless we have friends surrounding us like a firm wall against the winds of the world.
—*Charles Towne*

Friends can either sustain us or bring us down. We all have had friends who are negative and caustic. I am not saying to stop being their friend, but to limit how much time you spend with them.

We should strive to have friends who are that "firm wall against the winds." Unlike our family, we can choose our friends.

Remember that some friends are for a season, some for a reason, and some for a lifetime. Not all friends are meant to be in your life forever. Don't try to hold on if it's time for them to go.

But, just as with your significant other and co-workers, you must cultivate your friendships. Don't take them for granted. Remember to list your friends on your gratitude list that we talked about in chapter 3.

No matter what looms ahead, if you can eat today, enjoy today, mix good cheer with friends today, enjoy it and bless God for it.
—*Henry Ward Beecher*

Cultivate your relationships. You will be richer for it.

CHAPTER 15

YOUR PERSONAL PATHWAY TO PEACE AND TRANQUILITY

Thoughts from Mary Jo:

The search for a better quality of life has become the modern-day quest for the Holy Grail. Like medieval knights, we seek this seemingly elusive goal that we hope will bring everlasting happiness. In America, we spend millions of dollars a year on therapy in search of what will finally bring contentment to our unhappy or stressful lives.

Throughout human history, religions, philosophies, and cultures, we have attempted to promote a higher quality of life. Christianity, Judaism, Buddhism, Islam, Hinduism, the teachings of Plato, Confucius, Epicurus, and now modern science all promote a better way of living using surprisingly similar techniques. Unfortunately, many of us simply fail to practice these techniques or give up when the techniques do not lead to an immediate and constant state of happiness.

Regardless of what religion or philosophy you practice, all of these teachings show us how to be kind to others, focus less on our problems, appreciate what we have, and clear our minds of negative feelings through prayer and/or meditation. They also teach that life is not easy, but if you learn certain skills to help you with the difficulties of life, you can achieve contentment regardless of your prior pain.

Of course, the actual task of acquiring coping skills is hardly effortless. It requires learning how to discipline the brain to abandon negative thoughts and feelings. The problem lies not in having a negative thought, but in dwelling on it. Dwelling on negativity has become a bad habit for many of us and, like all bad habits, can be very difficult to break. Although it is impossible to keep negative thoughts from occurring, it is possible to keep them from recurring.

Many call this a spiritual life, or being in touch with a higher power, or communing with the divine within you. Whatever you choose to call it, for you to truly have a "healthy" life, we believe that, like brushing your teeth, you should utilize this skill every day. To be healthy we, as women, must cultivate our bodies, minds, and spirits. To not "exercise" any one of these would be falling short of our goal to be happy, healthy, and harmonious.[15]

So, what can we do to "exercise" the spirit? Everyone, of course, has to choose her own path, but the following are some examples of pathways I have recommended to my clients:

Meditation and Prayer

For many of us, when we think of meditation, we think of the yogi sitting motionless with his legs crossed in a lotus position for hours. While that is definitely one form of meditation, it is certainly not the only form and definitely is not practical for our everyday lives. So what do I mean by meditation? There are as many forms of meditation as there are birds in the air. To name just a few, there are:

- Different forms of Buddhist meditation
- Christian contemplation
- Different forms of Hindu meditation
- Judaism meditation
- New-age or secular meditation
- Guided meditation

Meditation can be used to achieve a higher state of consciousness; to obtain greater focus, creativity, or self-awareness; or simply to find a more relaxed and peaceful frame of mind. Diana Robinson stated it this way: "Prayer is when you talk to God; meditation is when you listen." According to the Dalai Lama, "Meditation is an instrument to increase our mental energy and mental sharpness or alertness."

Why Should I Meditate?

In the early 1970s, Herbert Benson, a young Harvard cardiologist who would not have dared to use the word "meditation," published a book entitled *Relaxation Response*. In it, he gave us our first glimpse from a scientific or medical point of view of why we should meditate. Meditation, we learned, actually can reduce blood pressure.

Then Dr. Richard Davidson and Dr. Jon Kabat-Zinn burst onto the scene, via their work with the Mind and Life Institute. The work that all of these men have done (and many others continue to do) in mind-body medicine is remarkable.

They learned that through meditation you can reduce anxiety, PMS, blood pressure, inflammation, and depression, and even began to see that you can create changes in your genetic makeup. Vipassna Meditation, Mantric Meditation, Mindfulness Meditation, Transcendental Meditation, Breath Focus, Kripala Yoga, Kundalina Yoga, Repetitive Prayer—all led to the same relaxation response, as reported in Dr. Benson's work.

We are learning that the health benefits are limitless. So, whether you seek a higher state of consciousness, a particular health benefit, or just a more relaxed and peaceful state of mind, meditation can offer big benefits.

How Do I Get Started?

There is no one way to meditate. Perhaps you go to a bookstore and buy a guided meditation CD. There are many types, from a visualization, to a scan of your body, to awareness of your breathing. Many practices require you to sit up, but if that is not for you, then lie down with your palms up.

There are walking meditations, where you will very slowly (preferably in a park or someplace beautiful) become keenly aware of every flower, bird, or bug. Or breathing meditations, where you concentrate on your breath.

To get started with any of these or others, I suggest reading the book *How to Meditate* by Lawrence LeShan, or going to www.PrimeForLife.net for a guided meditation (click on "Samples"). Or, as I mentioned, you can go to your local bookstore and buy a guided meditation CD. You might also read the article by Janice Gates entitled "Presence of Mind," published in the June 2009 issue of *Yoga Journal*.

When asked why meditation is important in our daily lives, the Dalai Lama said: "Mental attitude is so influential in daily life that when you wake up in the morning and your mind feels happy or fresh, the rest of the day is good even in the face of a problem. If your mood is dull, even small things may lead you to eventually 'burst.' So, you see, mental attitude is a very important factor in our daily lives."[16]

Yoga

Yoga is derived from the Sanskrit root *yuj*, meaning "to yoke," or link. It is the linking of the breath and movement. Like meditation, there are many, many forms of yoga. While in the West we see yoga as a form of exercise or stretching, in reality yoga incorporates not only the asanas (postures) but meditation as well.

Not only does a yoga practice give you all the benefits of movement that we discussed in part 2, but research such as Dr. Benson's shows that it helps with stress and all those illnesses that come with it.

There are many different kinds of yoga: hatha yoga, kundalini swara, Bikram yoga, and several more. Look for a yoga studio near you and try it out. Give it three tries before deciding whether you like it. If you don't like that particular kind of yoga, try a different one. For example, Bikram yoga is done at 104 degrees. All that heat may not be for you. Before you go to a studio, discover what kind of yoga is practiced there and do a little research on it.

See if that studio begins or ends the session with a meditation. If it does, you can kill two birds with one stone. For some, though, just going through the asanas is a meditation in and of itself.

Regular Practice of the Faith of Your Choice

There is some fascinating research regarding the connection between happiness and longevity and belief in God or practice of one's faith.

At a Royal Economic Society Conference, Professor Andrew Clark of the Paris School of Economics reported that his research revealed higher levels of life satisfaction in people who believe in God.[17] Additionally, he found that they were able to better cope with divorce or losing a job or other of life's struggles.

Professor Leslie Francis, from the University of Warwick, states that there is evidence that this higher "life satisfaction" may come from the increased purpose of life that believers have.[18] Further, Professor Clark's research revealed an interesting phenomenon—that even people who don't believe in God are happier when they live in communities where others have a strong belief.

Mark Holder, Ben Coleman, and Judi Wallace did a study of children ages eight through twelve and found that spirituality in children is a significant predictor of happiness.[19]

So, what does all of this mean for us? Professor Clark described it like this: "What we found was that religious people were experiencing current day rewards, rather than storing them up for the future."[20]

Maybe what we can take away from this, be it meditation, yoga, or practicing our faith, is that whether it is our belief in a higher power or awareness of experiences of that which is within us, having a spiritual life gives us a balance, a feeling of total well-being.

When we practice gratitude, compassion, and connectedness to others, we have a whole new vision of ourselves and those around us. In the words of the Dalai Lama, "We want happiness, the happiness that comes from within us—inexpensive, isn't it? A happiness and peace that nobody can destroy, steal, or take away. This inner peace is most precious. The basis of inner peace is love and compassion."

Remember the story of the anxious boy who went to his grandfather, a very wise man, and said, "I have this war inside of me. How can I stop it?" His grandfather said, "I know, my son, it is two wolves in you that are fighting. One is angry, hateful, and jealous, and the other is generous, loving, and compassionate." The little boy asked, "Which one wins?" The grandfather answered: "*The one that you feed.*"

Meditation, yoga, or practicing your faith are each about finding that part of you that calls out for peace and harmony, and feeding it.

CHAPTER 16

TAKE THE WORDS "I CAN'T" OUT OF YOUR VOCABULARY: The Road to Change

Thoughts from Mary Jo:

We teach our children things that we sometimes forget to implement in our own lives. It wasn't "The Little Engine That Can't."

This is not a new concept—people two thousand years ago knew that your thinking shapes your reality. Proverbs 23:7 reads, "For as a man thinks in his heart, so is he." In 400 BC, Socrates wrote, "There is no disease of the body apart from the mind."

Indulge me for a minute and let me share some things I have had to struggle to learn, even though I was obviously taught them as a child. It has been a long road to change.

Along the road I learned that you must be careful how you think, for your life is shaped by your thoughts. Your life is determined not so much by what life brings you, but by the attitude you bring to life. It is not determined so much by what happens to you, but by how you look at and think about what happens to you. Of course, environment colors your life, but you can choose the color it has.

The thoughts you live with, the images you cherish, the things you say to yourself habitually, the spiritual relationships you cling to—these are the ways you think and what determine your life. Your inward thinking determines your outward actions.

I would like to suggest two ways of thinking while on your road to change.

1. **Think "struggle" rather than "reward"**

   We always want to start the other way—what am I going to get out of this? We hesitate to do anything we can't get a return on by nightfall. There is very little in life that offers reward without effort, appreciation without contribution, or recognition without accomplishment.

2. **Think "mental" rather than "environmental"**

   It is so easy to blame our situation on environmental or inherited factors: "I can't lose weight because being overweight is in my genes; I can't work out because after I come home from work I have kids to feed." In reality, it is the way we look at the situation. We are stuck in "I can't."

   My father often told the story of Joe, who worked as a janitor for a prominent church. Joe was faithful, efficient, and dutiful in his work. However, the staff often would leave him notes of things they wanted him to do, but he never seemed to get those things done. The church manager finally fired him.

   Joe was resourceful and opened a business of his own, and after a few years expanded it to two more locations. He decided that in order to expand further, he needed to take out a loan. After reviewing his financial information, the bank was glad to loan him the money. When Joe went to finalize the loan, the loan officer asked him to sign the papers. Joe explained that he did not know how to read and write, so he did not know where to sign. He went on to say, "I never could read those notes they were leaving me at that church."

   Shocked, the loan officer said, "You have done so well! Imagine what you could have done if you could read and write." Joe responded, "I imagine I'd still be the janitor of that church."

TAKE THE WORDS "I CAN'T" OUT OF YOUR VOCABULARY

Joe didn't let illiteracy, or getting fired, or a life that was undoubtedly more difficult than the average American's, keep him from pursuing his dreams.

Be careful how you think—for your life is shaped by your thoughts.

William Pitt (a former prime minister of Great Britain) was terribly crippled, probably by arthritis. It was reported that when someone would tell him that something was impossible, he would raise one of his crutches and say, "What's impossible? I live on impossibilities."

Ultimately, it is the environment on the inside that counts, not the outside.

So, let's look at the habits of centenarians and how they have lived such a long life. They have certain traits in common: [21]

1. They have a strong group of friends.
2. They stay about the same weight their entire adult lives and are not obese.
3. Most do not smoke.
4. They drink alcohol in moderation or not at all.
5. They stay physically active.
6. They are willing to always learn new things.
7. They eat plenty of fruits and vegetables.
8. They tend to be optimistic and are willing to deal with change.
9. They do not dwell on negative emotions.
10. They rely on spiritual beliefs to deal with difficult times.

What are the things you can do to make those changes? I would suggest that you do three things:

1. Write down no more than two changes you want to make.

2. Have an action plan for how to achieve those changes.
3. Tell someone about your plan.

The act of writing it down gives you clarity of thought that you can continually refer to when you need a boost. The action plan gives you a specific road map of how to accomplish your change. Telling someone else makes you more likely to do it because it gives you someone to be accountable to.

Why no more than two changes? If you have too many, you may become overwhelmed and not complete any of them. Once you have accomplished those two, then you can add two more.[22]

Let me give you an example of a goal I have for myself.

Goal: To have greater bone density in my spine.

Action Plan: 1) Skip rope for two minutes a day.
2) Wear my weight vest a minimum of three days a week.

So, start a whole new system of thinking on your road to change and remember, "As you think in your heart, so are you."

FINAL WORDS FROM MARY JO

Jyotsna, Jan, Lu, Kristi, and I leave you with the words of Florence Rink, because they truly say it all: "Keep dancing!"

BODY MASS INDEX CHART

BMI (kg/m^2)	19	20	21	22	23	24	25	26	27	28	29	30	35	40
Height (in.)	Weight (lb.)													
58	91	96	100	105	110	115	119	124	129	134	138	143	167	191
59	94	99	104	109	114	119	124	128	133	138	143	148	173	198
60	97	102	107	112	118	123	128	133	138	143	148	153	179	204
61	100	106	111	116	122	127	132	137	143	148	153	158	185	211
62	104	109	115	120	126	131	136	142	147	153	158	164	191	218
63	107	113	118	124	130	135	141	146	152	158	163	169	197	225
64	110	116	122	128	134	140	145	151	157	163	169	174	204	232
65	114	120	126	132	138	144	150	156	162	168	174	180	210	240
66	118	124	130	136	142	148	155	161	167	173	179	186	216	247
67	121	127	134	140	146	153	159	166	172	178	185	191	223	255
68	125	131	138	144	151	158	164	171	177	184	190	197	230	262
69	128	135	142	149	155	162	169	176	182	189	196	203	236	270
70	132	139	146	153	160	167	174	181	188	195	202	207	243	278
71	136	143	150	157	165	172	179	186	193	200	208	215	250	286
72	140	147	154	162	169	177	184	191	199	206	213	221	258	294
73	144	151	159	166	174	182	189	197	204	212	219	227	265	302
74	148	155	163	171	179	186	194	202	210	218	225	233	272	311
75	152	160	168	176	184	192	200	208	216	224	232	240	279	319
76	156	164	172	180	189	197	205	213	221	230	238	246	287	328

ACKNOWLEDGMENTS

There are several people we need to thank, because without them this book would not have been possible.

Amy Hunt and Margaret Brown, editors extraordinaire – Jyotsna, Jan, Lu, Kristi, and I have been most fortunate to have your help.

Many thanks to Lyle Wilson, ND, Dipl. Ac., OSB – for your sage advice and support. Lu and I understand more about stretching (and about life in general) because of you.

Jeff Farrell – for allowing us to use Park Cities Yoga Studio for our stretch photos.

Nancy Pinnow – for filling in on a couple of the stretch poses.

Jeff Anderson – for your time and your photographic contributions. They help make our message clearer and easier to visualize.

Mike Androvett – for your guidance through this process.

Randy Raugh – for the lessons I have learned from you at Canyon Ranch about creating and (more importantly) "internalizing" an action plan – how to turn a general goal into a very specific reality.

I would be remiss if I did not thank my legal assistants, Lou Ann Womack and Jonathan Broom – on top of your already sixty-plus-hour work weeks, you have worked with endless changes over the past two years. Thank you for your time and effort.

Last but not least, my husband Mike – for your love, support, encouragement, and advice. I am afraid you have learned much more about menopause than you ever wanted to know! Thank you for your patience with the many, many hours I spent working on this project instead of being with you. I love you.

Mary Jo McCurley

ENDNOTES

[1] Snowdon, D: "Healthy aging and dementia: Findings from the Nun Study" *Annals of Internal Medicine* 139 (5 Part 2):450454, 2003.

[2] Epel, E., Blackburn, E. H., Lin, J., Dhabhar, F. S., Adler, N. E., Morrow, J. D., and Cawthon, R. M. (2004). "Accelerated telomere shortening in response to chronic stress," *Proceedings of the National Academy of Sciences*, 101, 17312–17315.

[3] *U.S. Department of Health and Human Services, Informal Caregiving: Compassion in Action.* Washington, DC: 1998, and National Family Caregivers Association, *Random Sample Survey of Family Caregivers, Summer 2000, Unpublished.*

[4] *National Alliance for Caregiving and AARP, "Caregiving in the U.S.,"* 2004.

[5] "C'mon Get Happy," *Runners World,* April 2007.

[6] http://www.cdc.gov/healthyweight/assessing/bmi.

[7] For example, www.calorie-count.com.

[8] *Strong Women, Strong Hearts* by Miriam E. Nelson, M.D.

[9] Ibid.

[10] American Heart Association.

[11] *What Happy Women Know* by Dr. Dan Baker.

[12] *The Female Brain* by Louann Brizemdine, M.D.

[13] *What Happy Women Know* by Dr. Dan Baker.

[14] "Divorce: Prevention, Survival, & Recovery." (Article by Mike McCurley and Mary Jo McCurley)

[15] "Improving Quality of Life." (Article by Mike McCurley and Kelly Burris)

[16] *All You Ever Wanted to Know from His Holiness the Dalai Lama on Happiness* by Rajiv Mehrotra.

[17] http://www.pse.ens.fr/document/wp200901.pdf; "Let us pray: Religious interactions in life satisfaction," by Andrew E. Clark and Orsolya Lelkes.

[18] "Prayer, personality and purpose in life among churchgoing and non-churchgoing adolescents," in L. J. Francis, M. Robbins and J. Astley, eds. *Religion, Education and Adolescence: international*

empirical perspectives, Cardiff, University of Wales, Press, 2005, pp 15-38 (ISBN 0-7083-1957-2).

[19] Mark D. Holder, Ben Coleman, Judi M. Wallace (2008). "Spirituality, Religiousness, and Happiness in Children Aged 8–12 Years," *Journal of Happiness Studies* DOI: 10.1007/s10902-008-9126-1.

[20] http://www.pse.ens.fr/clark/DeliverPress.pdf; "Deliver Us from Evil: Religion as Insurance," by Andrew Clark and Orsolya Lelkes.

[21] Georgia Centenarians Study, New England Study. Okinawa Study.

[22] *Prime for Life* by Randy Raugh provides an excellent resource for anyone who needs help turning a vague goal into an actual, "doable" plan.

Made in the USA
Charleston, SC
11 July 2010